Claude McClure, M.D.

METHODS OF TREATMENT

IN

POSTENCEPHALITIC PARKINSONISM

METHODS *of* TREATMENT *in* POSTENCEPHALITIC PARKINSONISM

By

HENRY D. VON WITZLEBEN

Elgin State Hospital, Elgin, Illinois

Preface by

THEODORE J. C. VON STORCH

Associate Professor of Neurology, Albany Medical College;
Attending Neurologist, Albany Hospital,
Albany, New York

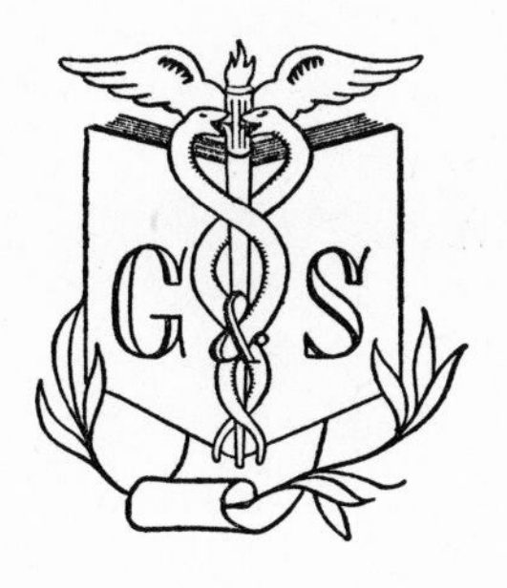

NEW YORK

GRUNE & STRATTON

1942

GRUNE & STRATTON, INC.
443 Fourth Avenue
New York City

Printed by
WAVERLY PRESS, INC.
U. S. A.

To the memory of the late

CONSTANTIN BARON VON ECONOMO

and to

FELIX STERN

this book is gratefully dedicated

CONTENTS

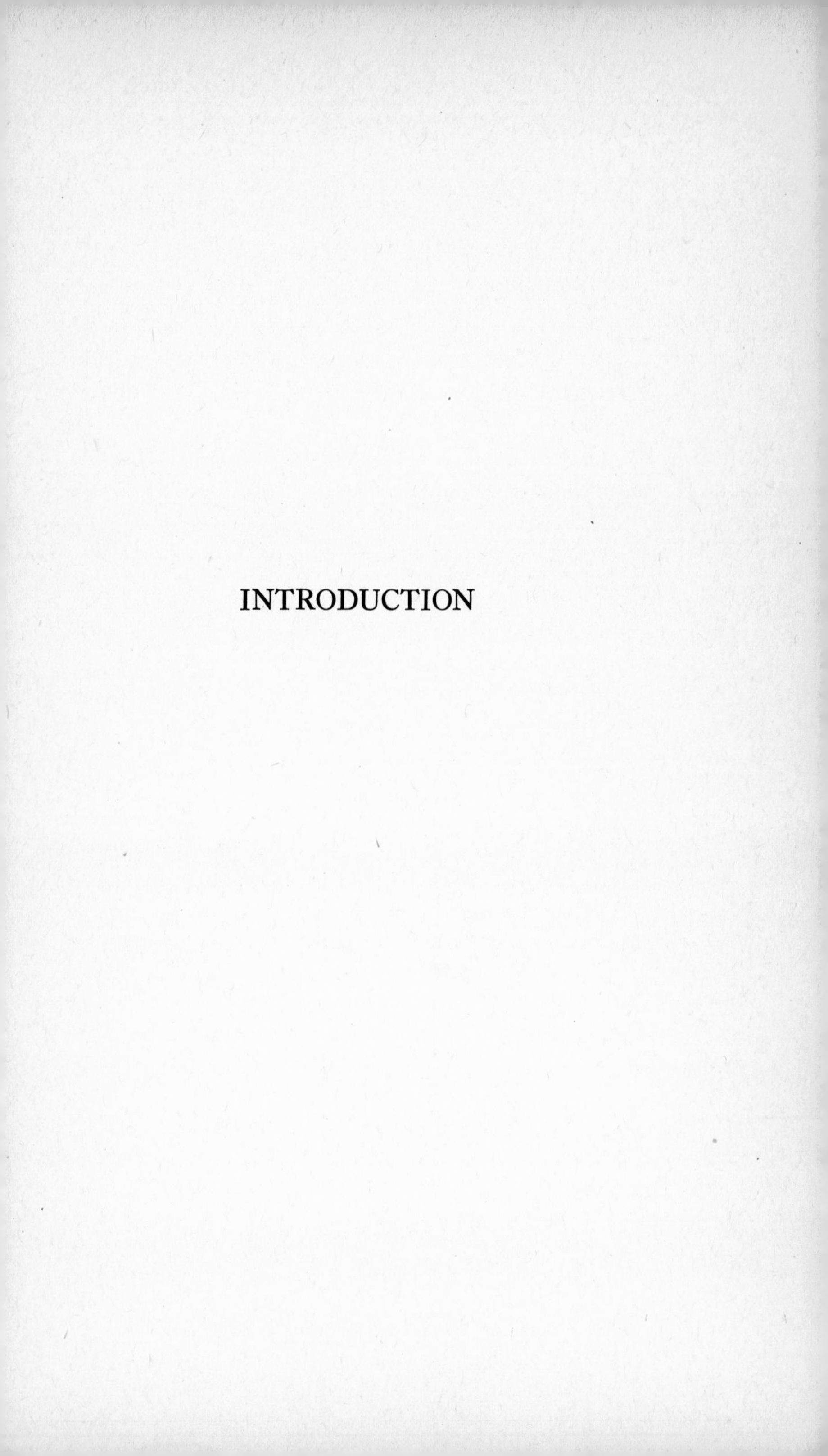

INTRODUCTION

INTRODUCTION

Doctor von Witzleben has already enriched the field of American medicine. His present monograph is another contribution to our knowledge and a progressive step in the control of postencephalitic Parkinsonism.

The author's extensive knowledge of this disease is based upon personal contact with hundreds of patients as well as upon a comprehensive study of the literature. His background of medicine at the Universities of Bonn, Freiburg and Berlin and of roentgenology at the Institute for Cancer Research at Heidelberg gives him a broad viewpoint for evaluation of various therapies. As assistant professor, associate professor, director and superintendent at several prominent institutes and hospitals for neuropsychiatric disorders, he has become familiar with the various aspects of neuropsychiatric treatment. In some thirty-three papers the author has contributed to many aspects of medicine, neurology and psychiatry. More than a third of these have been concerned with the nature and treatment of postencephalitic disorders.

The present monograph should be of much value to student, practitioner and specialist. The author has made a comprehensive review of the numerous therapies that have been recommended, with a brief evaluation of each. Many of these have now been discarded, others continue as a part of our present armamentarium. In the case of the more effective treatments, a practical description has been given. The most recent innovations cannot yet be evaluated. Quite naturally the author, who is an authority on the subject, has dwelt at length upon Bulgarian root treatment combined with physiotherapeutic measures. In his hands, as in others with similar patience and persistence, the results have been excellent in postencephalitic Parkinsonism.

The reader must be reminded that the first step in successful therapy is accurate differential diagnosis. To call all rigid, tremulous patients "Parkinsonians" is as illogical as to classify all those with convulsions as "epileptics." The author's chapter on differential diagnosis warrants careful study. After consideration, each case will fall into its proper category. Even then, however, each patient remains an individual therapeutic problem. Thoughtless application of various recommendations by the author may result in much disappointment. Proper use of the material in this book will, however, release many a patient from a life of imprisonment within himself.

THEODORE J. C. VON STORCH

Albany Medical College, 1942

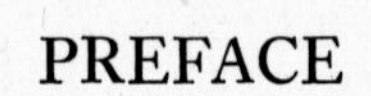
PREFACE

PREFACE

The literature concerning chronic postencephalitic Parkinsonism is voluminous, but no single compilation of the literature on therapy has yet been made. It has therefore been necessary to resort, painstakingly, to the original articles, in order to evaluate the various therapies recommended for this disease. One purpose of this book is to discuss, under one cover, all the forms of treatment that have been advanced. Another aim is to discuss the relative value of these therapies as seen in the light of the author's own experience. It is hoped that the resultant data may prove of value to the general practitioner as well as to the specialist in the field of neurology and psychiatry.

The large number of cases suffering from Parkinsonism poses an urgent social as well as medical problem. Reliable statistics on the frequency of the chronic disease do not seem to be available in any country, and in spite of the valuable assistance rendered by the governments of many countries, especially the Swiss Federal Health Department, I have been unable to secure definitive data regarding the number of patients suffering from this disease. It has been estimated by Panegrossi that about four individuals out of ten thousand suffer from this disease. Panegrossi's figures seem to be quite conservative, yet, if one accepts his estimate, more than sixty thousand persons are suffering from chronic Parkinsonism in the United States.

In dedicating this book to Constantin von Economo and to Felix Stern, I wish to express my deep appreciation and gratitude to the two men whose labors on the postencephalitic problem have been outstanding. Economo's first paper, published in 1917, in which he described all the ramifications of the clinical and therapeutic problems, is still the most important contribution on this subject. One is compelled, on reading this paper, to admire the keen observations made by the discoverer of encephalitis, considered to be the epitome of the Viennese Medical School which has long endowed the world with rich contributions.

Felix Stern has done a great deal of investigating and has made many excellent contributions to the encephalitic problem. It was due to his initiative that the first clinic devoted solely to the treatment of postencephalitic cases was established at the University of Göttingen. His monograph on postencephalitic Parkinsonism (Handbuch der Neurologie, Volume XIII) is masterly.

I should also like to express my thanks to the many colleagues who have helped me in the preparation of this volume, especially my former coworkers, Dr. M. Krueper and Miss R. Haufe, without whose indefatigable efforts it would have been much retarded. I am also grateful to Dr. Hans W. Maier, Director of the Psychiatric Institute in Zurich; Dr. M. Minkowski, Director of the Neurologic Institute, Zurich; and to Dr. P. J. Wolff of Buenos Aires, for their kind suggestions and the interest they have taken in this work. To Dr. Tracy J. Putnam of the Neurological Institute of New York, I wish to express my special thanks for his kind interest and assistance.

I wish to acknowledge my indebtedness to Dr. Theodore J. C. von Storch who has been very kind and helpful to me ever since my arrival in this country. In particular, I want to express my deep appreciation for the introduction to this book which he has written.

Acknowledgement is made to Dr. Stanley Cobb of Boston, Mass., to Dr. Clemens E. Benda, Wrentham, Mass., and to Drs. Charles F. Read, E. Liebert, and A. A. Lieberman, all of Elgin, Illinois, for their help in the preparation of this volume.

DIAGNOSIS AND DIFFERENTIAL DIAGNOSIS

Chapter I

DIAGNOSIS AND DIFFERENTIAL DIAGNOSIS

Since the beneficial effect of treatment depends not only on the severity of the clinical picture but also upon the underlying pathological process, it is extremely important that a definite diagnosis be established. Hence, a brief definition of the term "postencephalitic Parkinsonism" and a statement concerning the differential diagnosis appear imperative.

The term "postencephalitic Parkinsonism" has given rise to a great deal of misunderstanding, describing as it does the clinical picture but not depicting the underlying anatomical process. However, since the designation has been familiar to every physician for more than twenty years, it seems neither desirable nor necessary to coin a new word. But in adhering to the use of the term, the following extension of the definition is of fundamental importance. Postencephalitic Parkinsonism is not a sequela or a meta-disease of acute epidemic encephalitis, but is a form of chronic epidemic encephalitis typified by very characteristic signs.

The pathology consists of degenerative changes and scarring in cases of long duration, and of a progressive inflammatory reaction. This process is localized in the same regions in chronic forms as in acute epidemic encephalitis—in the basal ganglia, Luys' body and the substantia nigra. There are, in addition, true sequelae in postencephalitic Parkinsonism, which must be differentiated from the chronic progressive processes. Such sequelae manifest themselves as degenerations of the acute stage, as for example, paresis of muscles of the eye and paresis of accommodation. On the other hand, Stern's important, so-called "pseudo-neurasthenic stage" is almost certainly a sign of chronic encephalitis.

If postencephalitic Parkinsonism is a form of chronic epidemic encephalitis, it must be differentiated from all other forms of Parkinsonism, particularly from paralysis agitans, which is the original Parkinson's disease. Recently, Klaue has tried to show that there is no fundamental difference. But Hassler has clearly demonstrated that in postencephalitic Parkinsonism all groups of cells in the substantia nigra are altered, whereas in paralysis agitans only certain middle parts are involved. According to O. Vogt, the substantia nigra consists of two well-demarcated coextensive areas—the anterior and posterior parts. The former is connected with the striatum, the latter with the pallidum. The tremor in postencephalitic Parkinsonism is due to changes in the anterior part, while the rigidity is caused by lesions in the posterior part.

It cannot be denied that the clinical pictures of postencephalitic Parkinsonism and paralysis agitans often resemble each other; nevertheless, there are distinct features which differentiate the three most important forms of Parkinsonism—the postencephalitic type, the arteriosclerotic type, and paralysis agitans. Table I summarizes these features.

Postencephalitic Parkinsonism is characterized by a history of an episode of acute epidemic encephalitis, and inability to elicit a history of it does not necessarily exclude the possible occurrence of such an episode. However, an acute stage occurs only in postencephalitic Parkinsonism. In the experience of the author, age does not seem to be as significant as commonly affirmed. The interval between the acute disease and the first signs of Parkinsonism may fluctuate considerably, and there may be a free interval of seventeen years or more. Moreover, as the great epidemics of encephalitis become more distant in time, the age of the patient has less significance. Many patients now in the age group in which paralysis agitans is common show signs of postencephalitic Parkinsonism. This is not applicable to the same extent in the United States as in Europe, for during the last ten to fifteen years the incidence of acute cases of epidemic encephalitis has been considerably higher in the United States.

TABLE I

Comparison of the three principal types of Parkinsonism (Wilson)

	PARALYSIS AGITANS	ENCEPHALITIC PARKINSONISM	ARTERIOSCLEROTIC PARKINSONISM
Age at onset	Chief incidence 50–60	Any age from childhood: Mostly before 40	Old age
Onset	Gradual	Gradual	Sometimes rather quick
Course	Progressive and steady	Develops rather quickly: Often becomes stationary	Sometimes advances by exacerbations
Extent	May be partial, but becomes generalized	Parts affected often limited with little or no tendency to spread: May be generalized	Trunk and lower limbs principally
Type	Both rigidity and tremor frequent or nearly constant	Tremor exceptional, rigidity nearly constant	Almost entirely rigid, little or no tremor: Muscles feel hard
Accompaniments or complications	None	Other encephalitic residua: tics, spasms, respiratory disorders, behavioristic change etc. etc.	Pseudobulbar symptoms, forced laughing or crying, pyramidal signs, cortical symptoms (aphasia, apraxia etc.), evidence of arteriosclerosis
Special features	Dribbling and sialorrhea not very common, nor diplopia; pupil reactions good	Sialorrhea common, wet tongue, greasy skin over face, pupil reactions often impaired, diplopia usual	Cranial nerves much less affected in these ways, if at all: Senile myosis, perhaps

From Wilson, S. A. K. Neurology, Baltimore, 1940.

Rigidity, a characteristic of postencephalitic Parkinsonism, must be differentiated from spasticity, which occurs in various other disorders. Spasticity occurs predominantly in the flexors of the upper limbs and the extensors of the lower limbs. Upon stretching the limb, tonic resistance is maximal at the onset but decreases rapidly (clasp-knife rigidity). Spasticity, furthermore, shows the shortening and lengthening reaction (Sherrington) and is probably a proprioceptive reflex. Rigidity, on the other hand, is not predominantly confined to any special muscle group, but is diffuse in extent and equal in intensity throughout the movement. The following components of rigidity, which are described by O. Foerster, are of special value in differential diagnosis. They are: 1) Tremors, present during rest; 2) Increased plastic tonus; 3) Tendency to fixation of the muscle at whatever length is passively imposed upon it; 4) Tonic prolongation of the response to electrical stimulation; 5) Absence of irradiation of reflex movements and tonic prolongation of reflex response; 6) Absence of postural reactions during complex voluntary movements, and of expressional movements or when present, tonic prolongation of the latter; 7) Limitation of range, absence of spontaneity, slowness in imitation, and absence of normal associated movements in all voluntary movements.

Both postencephalitic Parkinsonism and paralysis agitans display a tremor. In postencephalitic Parkinsonism, however, the main sign is rigidity, quite often unaccompanied by any tremor, whereas in paralysis agitans the tremor is more prominent and appears earlier than rigidity. Absence of tremor, however, cannot be utilized as a strict differential feature in diagnosing postencephalitic Parkinsonism. Sometimes the tremor takes a phasic course, diminishing or disappearing for a time; but a potential tremor remains, which unfortunately often cannot be influenced by any treatment. The muscle must be in a certain tonic state for tremor to develop, since no tremors can occur in a flaccid atonic extremity. On the other hand, the more marked the rigidity, the less the tremor, which if it appears at all, is of very low amplitude. If the rigidity becomes diminished, as for example, by treatment, tremor may appear, or, if already present, become more obvious. A coarse tremor often occurs when rigidity is absent or not very marked. Proximal muscle segments which are markedly rigid show less tremor than peripheral segments, which are less rigid. These facts constitute one of the most interesting and difficult problems in any treatment of postencephalitic Parkinsonism, because of the close relationship between tremor and rigidity. As Hughlins Jackson has said: "Tremor differs from rigidity, not fundamentally but in degree." As he aptly phrases it, rigidity is "tremor run together."

Graphic recording of the tremor of paralysis agitans and of postencephalitic Parkinsonism shows no fundamental difference. Clinically, however, the two diseases show a difference in character. In paralysis agitans the distal ends of the upper extremity are especially affected, and pill rolling is present. Furthermore, it decreases upon intentional movements, whereas in postencephalitic Parkinsonism it is increased qualitatively and quantitatively by such movements. Gamper states that the pill-rolling tremor is characteristic only of paralysis agitans, while Stern and others, as well as myself, believe that this sign is seen also in postencephalitic Parkinsonism. In my own experience I have found it to occur in approximately 1 to 1.5 per cent of all cases. Passive stretching of the muscles in postencephalitic Parkinsonism results in rigidity and adaptational shortening. The tonus is normal at the beginning of the movement, increasing gradually and accompanied by an increased excitability of extension. Furthermore, in postencephalitic Parkinsonism tension without rigidity may occur.

Both Stern and Gamper state that the changes of muscle tonicity are of the same nature in both postencephalitic Parkinsonism and paralysis agitans, but are less intense in the latter. It is known that in postencephalitic Parkinsonism the first changes in muscle tonus appear in the muscles of the neck and face. The amimetic face is more marked in postencephalitic Parkinsonism than in paralysis agitans. Aphonia can be found in both diseases, but iteration, palilalia and bulbar phenomena seem to appear only in postencephalitic Parkinsonism, as do pareses of the eye muscles.

Contrary to the picture in paralysis agitans, that of the motor disturbances in postencephalitic Parkinsonism is more vivid and includes myoclonia, myotonia, tic, choreiform movement, athetosis, torsion spasm (dystonia musculorum deformans), complicated hyperkinesias of many different features, and oculogyric crises.

Cogwheel rigidity is an early sign in postencephalitic Parkinsonism and is much more pronounced than in paralysis agitans. Disturbances of chewing and swallowing also appear rather early and are apt to become quite serious. These disturbances are notably inconspicuous or absent in paralysis agitans, and are found only in the very advanced stages.

Moreover, in postencephalitic Parkinsonism vegetative disturbances are much more marked than in paralysis agitans; viz., attacks of perspiration, acrocyanosis, obesity or emaciation, disturbances in temperature regulation, marble-like discolorations of the skin of the lower extremities, and disturbances of sleep, mastication, heart functions and respiration. Bradyteleocinesia and often cataleptic signs are much more marked in postencephalitic Parkinsonism than in paralysis agitans. Panegrossi states that palilalia is absolutely pathognomonic for postencephalitic Parkinsonism.

There are no psychopathological features in paralysis agitans except for some general irritability and extremely rare compulsive phenomena, first described by Oppenheim in 1909. On the other hand, in postencephalitic Parkinsonism the bradyphrenia is very marked, and many other signs of mental disturbances are to be seen, ranging from simple psychopathic features to extremely severe psychotic states. One of the most important psychic characteristics is the unusual suggestibility of these patients.

In addition to the so-called bradyphrenia, we find compulsions and impulsions, inclinations to murder, and sexual delinquencies. In children and adolescents there are the well-known deviations in character and behavior. Hallucinations, paranoid ideas, catatonic states and states of cloudiness occur more often in postencephalitic Parkinsonism than in paralysis agitans and the "psychomotor limitation of the personality" (Bostroem) plays a great role in cases which are accompanied by obsessions, compulsions and impulsions.

At times it may be impossible to differentiate between a postencephalitic and a catatonic state. In such cases, one often succeeds by therapeutic trial or by administering 1 to 1.2 milligrams physostigmine, which accentuates all the symptoms and signs of Parkinsonism. This is especially valuable in causing a tremor that is otherwise latent. On the other hand, rigidity and tremor of nonencephalitic origin do not react to physostigmine.

If the sugar of the spinal fluid shows a rise to 90 to 120 milligrams per cent, one is probably dealing with a case of postencephalitic Parkinsonism. An extremely slow blood sedimentation rate is of far greater diagnostic significance than has hitherto been recognized (Stern-Piper). This reaction may be extremely prolonged, becoming especially so the longer the interval between the acute disease and the beginning of Parkinsonism. A slow sedimentation rate also indicates that degenerative rather than inflammatory processes prevail, and hence a not very good prognosis of response to nonspecific therapy.

Contrary to Klaue, the author believes that there are some additional signs in postencephalitic Parkinsonism and paralysis agitans which make differentiation between the two conditions possible. Increasing experience has convinced me of the inestimable value of the alkaloids, both in therapeutic effect and as a diagnosis ex juvantibus. Patients suffering from paralysis agitans tolerate only very small doses of Atropa belladonna or display early signs of intoxication. In my observation, these small doses have little or no therapeutic effect, and often aggravate the condition of the patient, whereas the opposite is true in postencephalitic Parkinsonism.

Although some of the differential signs are not always decisive, there is little doubt that in many cases a differential diagnosis is possible. The following main signs seem to me to be characteristic of postencephalitic Parkinsonism:

An acute stage of epidemic encephalitis
Intensive akinesia and deficiency of mimic and reactive movements
Frequent absence of tremor
Absence or infrequent appearance of pill rolling
Salivation
Oily skin
Supplementary complications, such as paresis of eye muscles, oculogyric crisis, sleepiness or sleeplessness
More pronounced mental disorders than in paralysis agitans
Remarkable improvement with Bulgarian treatment, for example Bulgakur.

The foregoing leads me to the conclusions that so-called postencephalitic Parkinsonism is a form of chronic epidemic encephalitis (Economo's disease), and that it is distinct from paralysis agitans (Parkinson's disease). The two diseases may be differentiated etiologically, clinically and pathologically. Careful investigation, examination, and analysis show distinctive signs which justify such a differentiation. Treatment with extracts of the roots of Atropa belladonna, the so-called Bulgarian treatment, makes such a differentiation obvious.

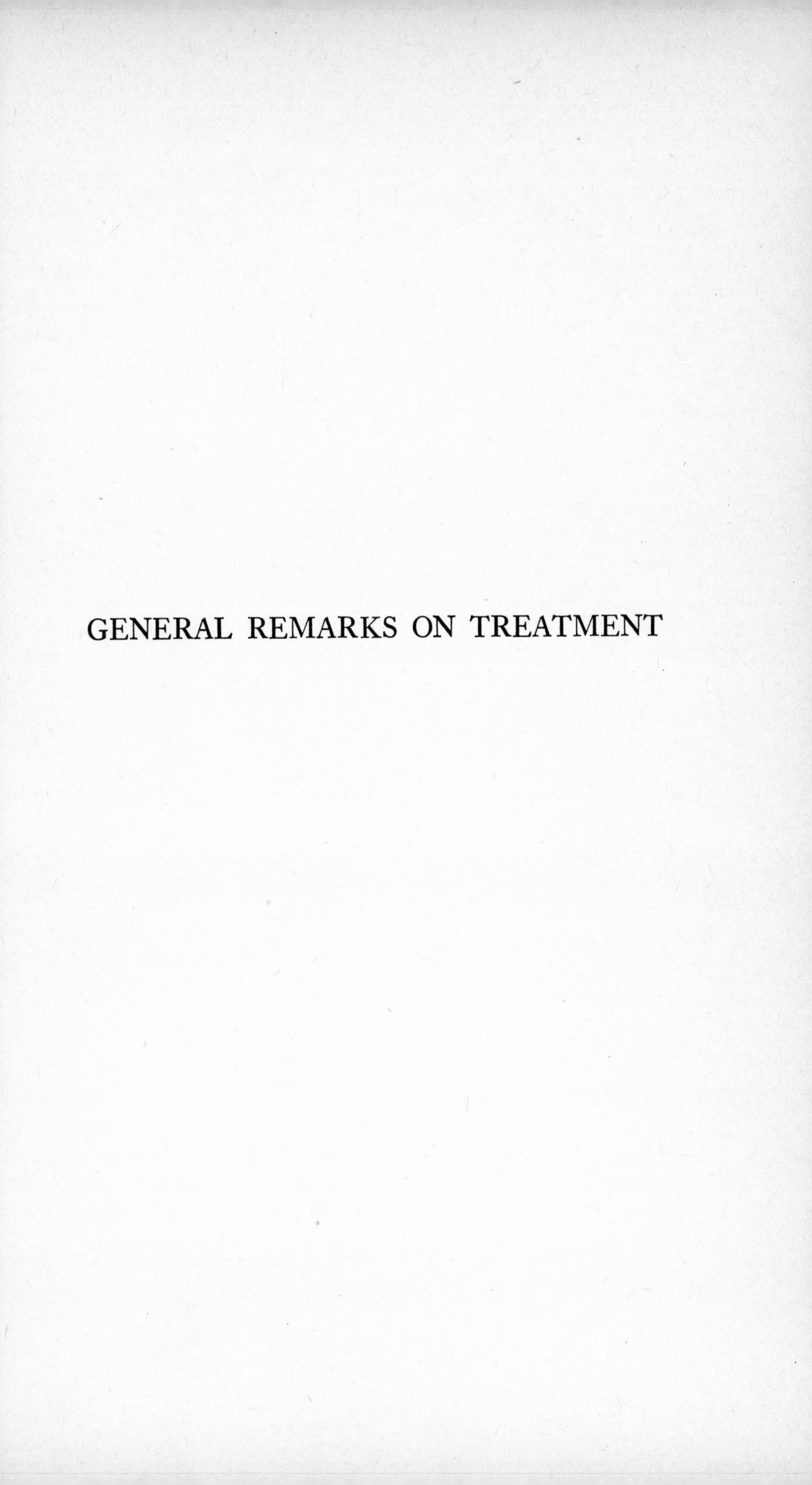

GENERAL REMARKS ON TREATMENT

CHAPTER 2

GENERAL REMARKS ON TREATMENT

Prior to the modern introduction of alkaloids in the treatment of postencephalitic Parkinsonism, it was considered relatively unamenable to therapy. Fleck and Rustige give an interesting report on the progress of 197 patients who were treated before the use of large doses of atropine had been introduced. The condition of most of the patients became worse and they were finally bedridden. Table 2 shows the working ability of these patients. Since the inception of alkaloid treatment, especially the combined method of the Bulgarian treatment, the results have become strikingly better, and at times are almost incredibly so.

It would seem that not only physicians, but also insurance companies and public and private welfare agencies ought to be much more interested in the treatment of these patients, who are often neglected and a burden to themselves and to society. There is no doubt that with the newest methods of treatment, a large percentage of these cases could be cured to a point at which they could resume work. A program similar to the one enacted in Italy in 1936 would be to the economic advantage of state and private hospitals. Several years ago O. C. Perkins proposed a similar program in New York. Ever since I have begun my work with encephalitics, a program which would permit such patients to be treated for a few months in a special ward of a hospital, by a staff specially trained for the work, has seemed advisable to me. Cases of postencephalitic Parkinsonism do not properly belong in a ward of psychotics; even when such a patient becomes psychotic, he still needs special attention and isolation from the quiet patients. Apart from the difficulties of treating patients suffering from postencephalitic Parkinsonism in a general ward, the atmosphere of such a ward has a deleterious influence upon these patients. One should not forget that in spite of many mental disturbances and psychomotor deviations in personality, a large part of the psychic life of these patients functions normally. Even though they are unable to express what is going on within them, there *is* an inside and they *have* an emotional and effective life, often a very sensitive one. A special encephalitic ward for handling excited and combative patients would also be advisable. Last but not least, such a segregation of postencephalitics would facilitate research work which, as Perkins pointed out in his article, is impossible in the surroundings of the ordinary ward.

TABLE 2

	MALE	FEMALE	PER CENT
Not able to work before and after treatment	112	55	86.6
Partly able to work before and after treatment	6	11	6.8
Markedly and continuously improved after treatment	4	9	6.6
Total	122	75	
	197		

The creation of such an encephalitic unit at a state hospital is not too difficult. It could then serve as a center for the treatment of all chronic encephalitics, and it could easily become the center for research on the clinical, pathological and biochemical problems of chronic encephalitis. The ideal unit would be equipped with all modern facilities, including a pool for underwater treatment, baths, a hall for calisthenics, a garden, rooms for occupational therapy, and so forth.

It need hardly be pointed out that before treatment is started a thorough physical and mental examination must be made. In women, pregnancy, always a serious complication in postencephalitic Parkinsonism, must not be overlooked, as it aggravates the patient's condition and almost always ends in the death of mother and child. Postencephalitic Parkinsonism, therefore, always constitutes an indication for therapeutic abortion, and when the proper medico-legal responsibility can be secured, sterilization should be performed.

During the general physical examination, sources of focal infections, such as teeth and tonsils, should be investigated. It has not yet been established whether such infections are of any etiological importance. While Eschke and Hempel report that very occasionally some infectious diseases are followed by a Parkinsonian state, no such case has occurred in my own experience. Otto Meyer states that latent phlebitis, to which he has called attention for many years, also plays a role in the etiology of postencephalitic Parkinsonism. I myself have seen neither this, nor the irritability which presumably follows pressure on the jugular vein, and which Meyer describes as typical. In any case, if such infections are present, they should be removed, whether they are of etiological importance or not, as they may be followed by very undesirable and dangerous complications.

Careful attention should be given the general physical condition, as the indications for various methods of treatment may depend upon it. If, for example, a slight hyperthyroidism is overlooked and iodine is administered, a very disagreeable iodine intoxication may occur. When the patient is in poor physical condition, emaciated and losing weight, he must be carefully observed for several days before any treatment is started. Diet is also important and should be regulated according to the needs and peculiarities of the patient. The diet should be rich in vitamins, and should contain little meat, but much fruit and vegetables. Fuch's acid diet seems to be without any value.

It has seemed advisable to me to abandon Panegrossi's rule forbidding any meat. This prohibition, which is perhaps reasonable in Italy because of the effect of climate, does not seem useful elsewhere. Nevertheless, some restriction of the meat consumption seems to be desirable. This can be done by allowing meat twice a week.

It is wise to limit the patient to one cigar or two to three cigarettes a day. This is better than forbidding tobacco completely, in view of the difficulty of enforcing complete abstinence. Therapeutically, however, complete abstension from the use of tobacco, as advised by Freeman, seems to me to be best. If tobacco is to be withheld from the patient, it should be done before treatment is begun, in order to avoid the appearance of withdrawal symptoms occurring simultaneously with the introduction of alkaloids.

Whatever concessions in the use of meat and tobacco must be made, none at all should be made in regard to the use of alcoholic beverages. Not even the smallest amount should be allowed, and the restriction should include beer and new wine, which many European patients do not consider as alcoholic beverages. I have found the effect of alcohol to be so deleterious that I have been rigidly unyielding in enforcing complete abstinence from it. I have seen severe psychotic excitement and agitation to follow the consumption of as little as half a glass of beer.

It does not seem to me to be necessary to forbid tea and coffee—as Panegrossi believes—provided that they are consumed in small quantities and in weak concentrations.

The question of rest and exercise is an important one and not at all easily managed. The patient himself is inclined to "have a rest," to do nothing, or to dawdle about. Such "treatment" is abundantly furnished in institutions, which devote small attention to and provide little stimulation for these people. This is however the worst sort of "treatment." While overexertion and excessive fatigue are to be avoided, a reasonable "total push" treatment can do little harm. The progressive lethargy of limbs can be avoided by daily massage and calisthenics, as well as by occupational therapy, walking or playing. The body tolerance to exercise must be evaluated for each patient, and short periods of rest inserted. This rest is preferably taken out of doors, but care should be taken to avoid exposure to direct sunlight, as postencephalitic patients are hypersensitive to heat and irradiation.

The advantages of such a strict division of the day should not be underestimated. The patient soon realizes gratefully that a well-considered program has been planned, not merely to keep him occupied or to pass the time, but one which is also beneficial to him. One seldom encounters any resistance on the part of the patient; on the contrary, patients take to this bodily and mental discipline which they soon discover contributes to their well-being. A discipline which becomes the main foundation of the proper and adequate management of the patient during and after his hospital stay seems to me to be of vital importance. If the patients have learned what to do for themselves, almost all of them will continue to do so, and thus succeed in making a good adjustment at home. The lack of such training and the difficulty in introducing it constitutes, in my opinion, the main reason for the much less favorable results from the treatment of postencephalitic Parkinsonism in outpatient departments of hospitals or in the practitioner's office. According to Vollmer and other authors, the treatment in a hospital with all its facilities, the daily discipline, and the removal from home and worries are *the* essential factors which have complicated the proper evaluation of treatment with the extract of belladonna root. This conception, in my opinion, arises from a misunderstanding of the basic principles. Proper hospital care is merely an important adjunct in the treatment of Parkinsonism. The patient suffering from postencephalitic Parkinsonism should not be brought to the hospital merely to enjoy the efforts of others on his behalf, but he himself must be encouraged to cooperate and to learn a very strict discipline. The *milieu* of the hospital, therefore, may be considered a *training milieu* which, together with certain methods of medical and physical treatment, will improve the patient's state. Neither the stay in the hospital alone, nor the medical or physical treatment alone are able to produce satisfactory results, but only the correctly applied combination of all of them.

As in many other disorders which are resistant to ordinary methods of treatment, the use of various vitamins has been recommended. Jolliffe and Spies have both used vitamin B_6 hydrochloride (pyrodoxin) because of its effect on muscle metabolism. They have reported objective and subjective improvement in six out of ten early cases of postencephalitic Parkinsonism, which they treated by intravenous injection of 50 to 100 milligrams of vitamins daily or every other day. Further observations are necessary to substantiate these views. Gangl and Lucksch report one case of postencephalitic Parkinsonism with oculogyric crises which, though resistant to atropine, was improved for two months, after ten injections of a vitamin C preparation (Cantan).

Treatment with large doses of arsenic, as recommended by the French, can be considered only as a tonic measure, similar to the use of iron or strychnine. It is indicated in cases of exhaustion and emaciation. The French are inclined to administer a 50 per cent solution of sodium cacodylate intravenously, starting with 0.2 to 0.5 cc. and increasing the dose every third or fourth day up to 2 to 5 cc., giving a total of 50 to 80 cc. The interval between injections should be five to six days, because of retarded excretion from the body. Although French authors report a decrease in rigidity and tremor produced by a mild arsenic neuritis, like Katona, I have noted improvement only in the general condition, such as added weight and better mood.

Neosalvarsan was tried by Agostini, his dose being 0.15 to 0.5 grams once a week. However, its use seems to me to be contraindicated because of the possible dangerous effect on a brain already impaired by a serious disease.

In cases complicated by anemia, liver preparations are of greater value than iron; and the combination of liver and arsenic is a very good one.

Froment has administered 8 to 10 milligrams of strychnine,

as he believes that the extrapyramidal hypertony is due to an insufficiency in the static posture mechanism. In my experience, strychnine has been found useful in cases displaying narcolepsy and cataleptic attacks following emotional upsets. Hermann has obtained good results by giving pills of 0.0002 grams twice daily.

The so-called organic therapy (Striaphorin and other preparations) of Cohn, Enge, Weiss and Rosin is of little importance.

According to Fawcitt, treatment with ultraviolet rays may be of considerable help, especially because it influences sleep. Irradiation should be done twice a week, for ten to twenty minutes, at a distance of 40 centimeters. After six to seven weeks, a new course of treatment is begun. This treatment may be considered as a tonic measure.

Froment and his collaborators introduced the treatment of postencephalitic Parkinsonism with insulin. It is their belief that a considerable acidosis exists, and that the decreased alkali reserve is raised to the normal level by insulin, while at the same time the increased basal metabolism returns to normal. Froment gave 10 to 15 units daily, and noted a salutary influence on the cachexia and, when used together with hyoscine, upon the rigidity. He has also used, in postencephalitic narcolepsy and states of depersonalization, 5 units daily, reporting excellent results. My own experience in its use is limited, and I have never seen any remarkable effects to result from the use of insulin in postencephalitic Parkinsonism. Insulin, however, is useful with regard to the general bodily condition.

Believing that the increased sugar in the spinal fluid constitutes a good medium for Wiesner's gram-negative diplococci, Arghiris proposed the combination of insulin with urotropine. The theoretical basis of this treatment is inadequate and the Wiesner diplococcus is without etiologic importance.

Staehelin described a case of postencephalitic Parkinsonism with acoustic, optic, and sensory hallucinations, in whose family there were several cases of schizophrenia. The patient was treated with insulin for four weeks, being given 85 to 130 units, and had two light and thirteen severe phases, and deep shock on eight occasions. Following this treatment, the patient became worse and his hallucinations were aggravated. However, the response of this one case cannot be considered as typical. As already mentioned, it is sometimes very difficult or impossible to determine whether one is dealing with a case of schizophrenia or Parkinsonism, or with a schizophrenic who also suffers from Parkinsonism. However, there would seem to be no reason why insulin therapy or electric shock treatment should not be used in similar cases, where contraindications do not exist.

The use of metrazol does not appear to be indicated, although Ziskind and Sommerfeld have treated a case with severe oculogyric crises, but without psychosis, with five injections of 5 cc. each. The patient had five severe epileptic seizures, after which he improved markedly, gained weight, the crises were diminished, and his mood became euphoric. However, the treatment had no effect whatever on the rigidity.

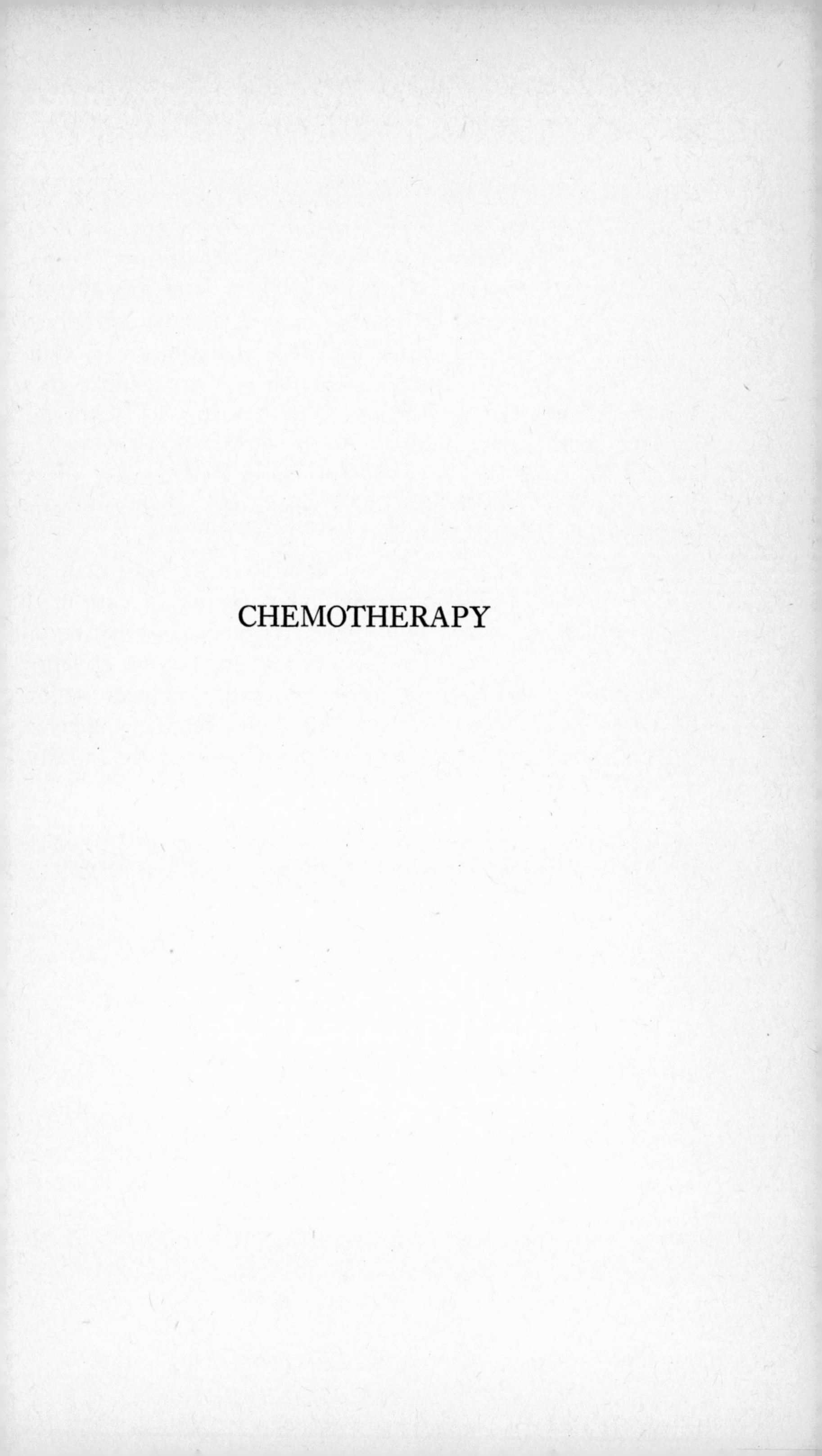

CHEMOTHERAPY

Chapter 3

CHEMOTHERAPY

As is common in the management of obscure diseases, many different chemical remedies are employed in the treatment of postencephalitic Parkinsonism. The basis of this treatment is Ehrlich's concept of therapia sterilisans magna, i.e., the attempt to destroy or attenuate the bacillus. The classic method of iodine treatment was introduced by Economo, and is combined with urotropine and vaccineurin (a nonspecific protein). This treatment is given in both the acute and chronic states, as Economo believes that cases energetically treated during the acute stage have a greater chance of escaping postencephalitic Parkinsonism. He feels that every case of postencephalitic Parkinsonism should be treated as if it were an acute one and should be given a course of treatment twice a year.

The treatment begins with the intravenous injection of vaccineurin, which is readily tolerated in Parkinsonism. The original solution is diluted with 0.9 per cent saline solution. Initially 1 cc. of 1 part of the original solution to 250 parts of sodium chloride is administered. Succeeding solutions are given in the following dilutions: 1:200; 1:150; 1:100; 1:50; 1:25; 1:20; and 1:10. Twelve injections are given in all, one every other day, together with 1 to 2 grams of urotropine daily. On an average the temperature remains in the vicinity of 39.5°C. (103°F.).

In the use of Pregl's iodine solution, which is similar to Lugol's solution, a trial injection of 20 cc. is given to discover a possible idiosyncrasy. It is followed on the succeeding day by 50 cc., injected intravenously, 100 cc. two days later, and thereafter 100 cc. three times a week up to a total amount of

1,000 to 2,000 cc. The injections injure the veins, but a freshly prepared solution will do so less than a stale one. As the brown solution is unstable when exposed to daylight, it must be stored in dark bottles. Old solutions which have turned yellow should be discarded. Septojod is an iodine solution ten times stronger than Pregl's solution. Only 10 to 15 cc. are used for each intravenous injection. I have found it better to use septojod, since, containing less free iodine, it injures the veins only slightly and causes no thrombosis, though large doses may seriously injure the retina. Heart diseases are a contraindication to its use. Sodium iodide may also be tried—20 cc. of a 33 per cent solution, two to three times a week—but not potassium iodide. According to Economo, potassium iodide is very dangerous and should be avoided, as it has a deleterious effect on the heart. It seems to me, therefore, that the treatment recommended by Olsen—50 to 100 cc. of a 10 per cent solution, several times a week—should not be used. All the more so, as Olsen himself reports the occurrence of fever and convulsive-like states. If one wishes to use Klemperer's solution (a 10 per cent solution of sodium iodide in water), 100 cc. once a week should be given, up to a total of ten to fifteen injections.

Iodine treatment yields the best results in those cases in which the inflammatory process prevails over the degenerative one. If the blood sedimentation rate is very slow, giving evidence of the prevalence of degeneration, hope for success is slight. There can be little doubt that iodine therapy is nonspecific. In my own experience, the results of this method have been modest. There may be cases which can be treated successfully, first with iodine and vaccineurin, and later with belladonna extract, but my own material is too scant to judge of that.

As mentioned previously, many chemical preparations have been tried, but most of them warrant little comment at this time. Many recommend the intravenous injection of 0.1 gram trypaflavine in 20 cc. of distilled water, every other day. After six injections, an eight-day rest period is allowed, after which treatment is started again, but increasing the amount of each injection to 0.2 gram in 20 cc. of water. Marx states that out of forty cases, fourteen improved markedly and twenty-two slightly, while four severe cases were influenced favorably. The improvement in eleven cases persisted, while the remainder became worse. I myself have discontinued the use of trypaflavine, after noting adverse general and skin reactions and the absence of any effect upon the Parkinsonian state. In one case, hypersensitivity to light became so pronounced that the patient had to be kept in darkness for a few days. This experience confirms an opinion long held by me, and expressed many years ago in an article on the X-ray treatment of mental and nervous diseases, namely, that postencephalitics are extremely sensitive to iodine, trypaflavine, salvarsan, and X-rays.

Unlike Agostini, who advises the use of salvarsan in doses of 0.15 to 0.5 gram, once a week, I do not find the use of this drug advisable, particularly in view of the cerebral sequellae in a brain already injured by a serious disease.

Inhalation of amyl nitrate is supposed to diminish oculogyric crises (Aymés). But amyl nitrate, of course, can only be administered for short intervals, and cannot be employed continuously.

One of the oldest remedies in medicine, mercury, may have some favorable effect, but in general it has not lived up to expectations. Paasche and others have tried injecting a 1 per cent solution of mercuric cyanide, 1 cc. every other day, to a total of 20 cc., giving a second series after an interval of ten to fourteen days. Ornstein and Orestianu report the improvement of one case in sixteen! I have always regarded this method as dangerous and in its stead have applied the time-proven inunction which is milder in action and of more uniform effect. Its application is identical in technique to that employed in the treatment of syphilis (up to 5 grams daily). Not every case can be treated with mercury, but it is useful and may produce sustained improvement in those cases which show increased intracranial pressure due to inflammation and adhesions of the meninges. However, I have never observed any significant effect upon rigidity or tremor. During its use, strict hygiene of the mouth must be observed, and the urine should be carefully examined.

Antimony is without value. Silvestri's report is open to criticism; he treated one case and obtained a restitutio ad integrum! Stibenyl was given uninterruptedly for as long as nine months without the slightest effect.

Carnot and Barry were the first to use salicylates, noting a specific effect. However, though for many years salicylates have been known to have a favorable influence on tremor when it is present without rigidity, to judge from the results obtained by Epstein, Farnham, and Cobb, there can be little doubt that salicylates have neither a specific nor any other effect in Parkinsonism. These authors administered 31 grains of a 20 per cent solution of a pure, crystallized preparation, intravenously. Three cases out of twelve showed some improvement for a short time, but later became worse.

Laignel-Lavastine and Sterne suggest the use of trypan blue and state that the rigidity became somewhat ameliorated in fifteen cases treated with this preparation. Chevallier, Schwob, and Durandy gave 1 to 6 cc. of a 1 per cent solution intravenously in one case, with the same result. McCartan reports uniformly unsatisfactory results.

Russetzki has demonstrated that magnesium chloride decreases muscle tone. Billigheimer has verified the diminution in tonus. Santangelo has employed magnesium sulfate combined, however, with hyoscine and iodine. On the whole, the results have not been noteworthy.

Potassium permanganate is recommended by Dejanoff, who injects 0.2 to 1.0 grams, in a solution of 1:1,000, in increasing doses every other day, up to fifteen injections. Gamarnik has seen improvement in eleven out of thirteen cases. While the injections are not dangerous, they are exceedingly painful. Sepp and others have created a so-called oxytherapy, which consists of injecting 300 cc. of oxygen into the thigh; the emphysema disappears within two days. At the same time, oxygen is inhaled three times a day, and in addition 1 cc. of a 1 per cent solution of potassium permanganate is given intramuscularly every other day. This treatment presumably exerts a beneficial influence on the general metabolism, and, in addition, the movements become quicker. If used at the very onset of the disease, it is said to arrest its progress.

Schacherl has administered calcium, giving it twice weekly as a mixed injection of calcium, 0.02 gram parathyroid, vaccineurin, and sodium cacodylate. It cannot, however, be recommended.

The results of chemotherapy are not encouraging. The only treatment of value is the original iodine-vaccineurin method introduced by Economo. Furthermore, mercury inunctions should be tried in any case which shows a high spinal fluid pressure due to inflammatory processes, such as adhesions of the meninges, blocking of one or more ventricle, and so forth.

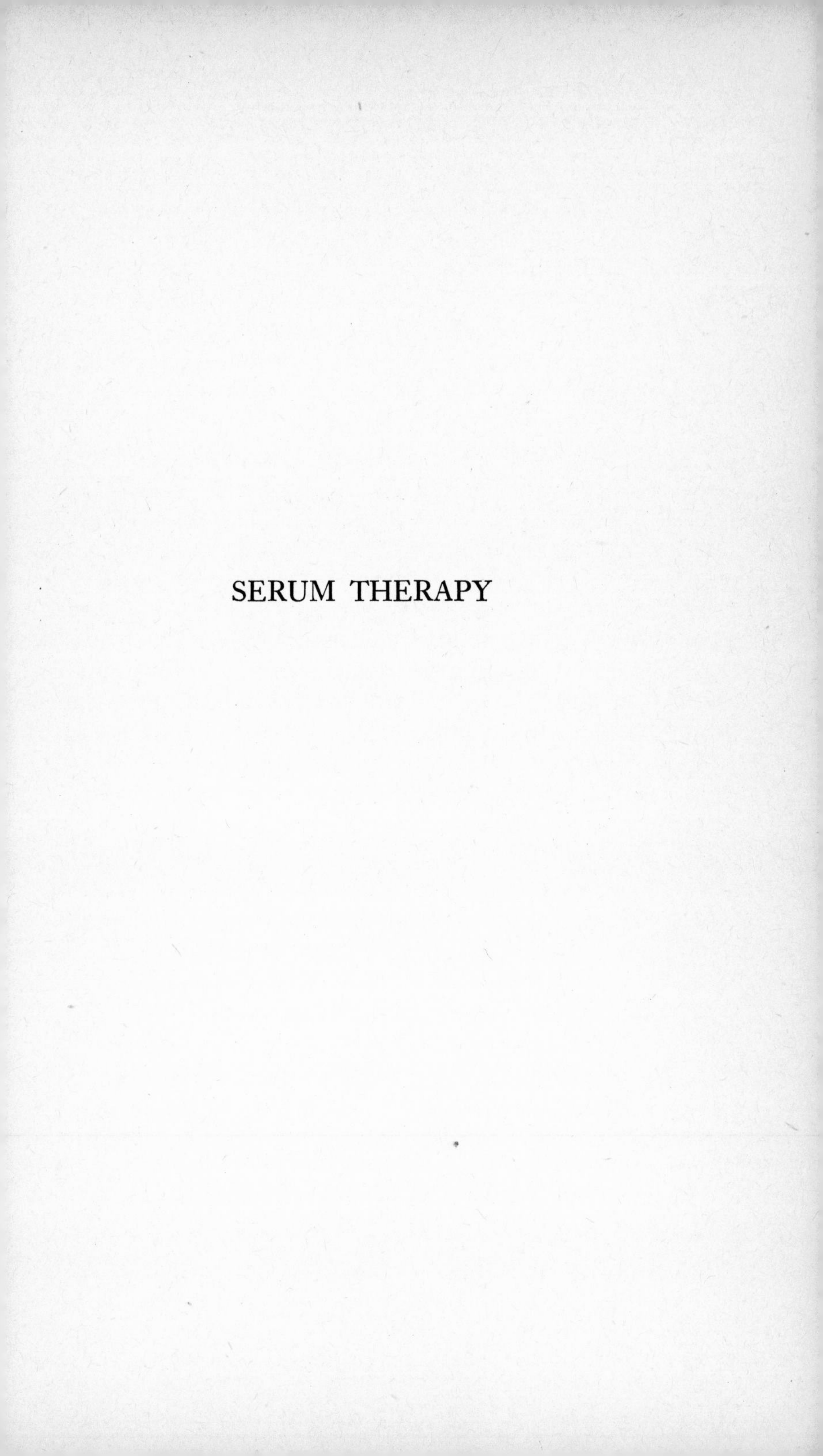

SERUM THERAPY

Chapter 4

SERUM THERAPY

Felix Stern was the first to describe the efficacious use of convalescent serum in acute cases of epidemic encephalitis. However, its effect in postencephalitic Parkinsonism is negligible, and I am in agreement with J. B. Neal that the use of convalescent serum seems particularly unjustified, in view of the fact that "so many patients fail to produce sufficient antibodies to check the course of the disease in themselves." Moreover, convalescent serum is obviously rare and should be saved for acute cases only. The attempts by Sicard and by Souques to stimulate autogenous antibody formation by injecting the patient's own spinal fluid intravenously failed completely, and Piticarin's case (only one) is not sufficient to alter this opinion. Dejanov noted temporary improvement after injection of nonspecific serum (horse serum) and Rosenthal was satisfied with a polyvalent grippe serum which was injected intramuscularly, 10 cc. being given the first day, 20 cc. the third, and 30 cc. the fifth day. The first injection brought sharp improvement which was maintained for several months. If the patient becomes worse, he recommends that the series be repeated, but that ox-serum be used in the second series, to avoid possible anaphylactic shock. My own experience has been limited to convalescent serum, with uniformly negative results.

Rosenow's encephalitis antistreptococci serum has not measured up to expectations. To obtain the serum, he isolated a peculiar streptococcus from the tonsils, teeth, and nasopharynx of patients suffering from epidemic encephalitis, which, inoculated into animals, produced typical symptoms of encephalitis.

The serum obtained from these animals was administered to patients with postencephalitic Parkinsonism by injecting hypodermically 0.5 cc. two to three times within twenty-four hours, followed by 20 to 40 cc. intravenously, or intrathecally! The results obtained from two cases seem doubtful and poorly controlled; the rationale likewise appears questionable. It has not yet been proven, as Rosenow seems to believe, that epidemic encephalitis is caused by a neurotropic streptococcus.

It is Gay's concept that the cause of encephalitis is a neurotropic strain of an herpetic-like virus. He has succeeded in producing a hyperimmune rabbit serum, but its efficacy awaits further testing and experience. Stewart and Evans have tried a soluble antigen and the immune horse serum of the Pfeiffer bacillus, but found no improvement in the rigidity of the patient.

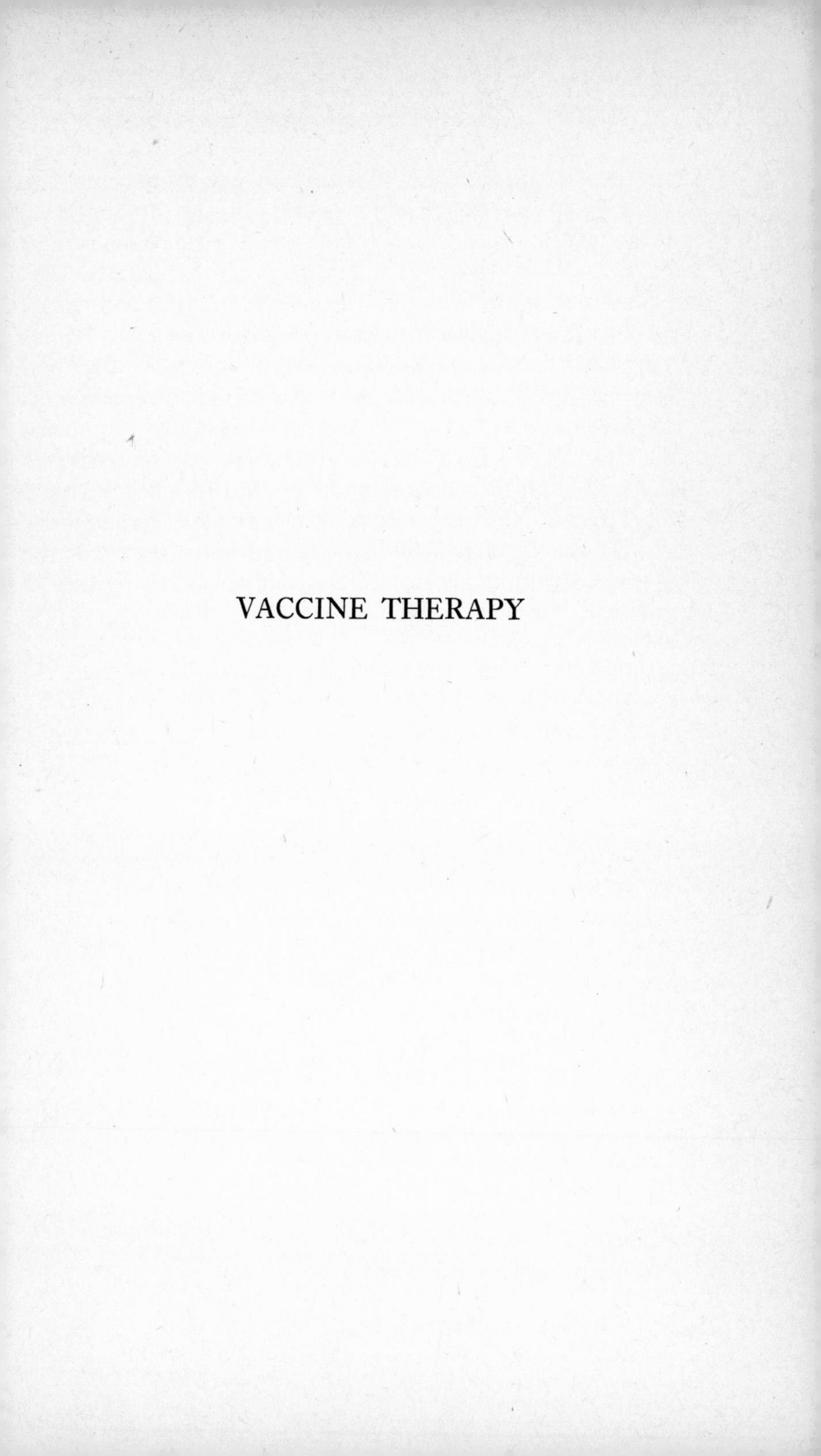

VACCINE THERAPY

Chapter 5

VACCINE THERAPY

Abraham and Victor have used influenza vaccine (soluble antigen of the Pfeiffer bacillus) in 125 cases. Though the patients were treated for as long as eighteen months, there were no results. Stewart and Evans employed the vaccine of the Hammett strain of the Pfeiffer bacillus.

Stransky gave typhoid vaccine together with 0.2 gram of sodium caffeine benzoate, basing his treatment on the rationale that since caffeine accelerates the metabolism of the tissues, the infective toxins are more quickly eliminated. He purports to have had satisfactory results. I myself have had no experience with this treatment.

There are two main theories in regard to the etiology of epidemic encephalitis: 1) Epidemic encephalitis may be caused by a form of a herpes virus (Levaditi); 2) It is caused by a neurotropic form of the streptococcus viridans (Rosenow, Evans and Freeman). Although in our present stage of knowledge we must question the validity of the former theory, treatment along these lines is not always devoid of value. Levaditi injected, intracerebrally, the virus obtained from a case of epidemic encephalitis into a group of rabbits, who recovered after having shown symptoms of encephalitis. The brains were emulsified, then sterilized and used as a vaccine. He also injected this vaccine intrathecally. Levaditi, Marie, Fournier, and Schwarz reported favorable results whereas le Fèvre de Arric and Sicard failed to observe any effects. Levaditi states that a rise in temperature is necessary to insure an effect. The effect is supposed to be nonspecific.

In the Neurological Institute in New York, Dr. Neal used

vaccine F, consisting of a formalized virus of a neurotropic herpetic-like type. The vaccine is prepared by inoculating rabbits intracerebrally with the virus, removing the brain at the height of illness and then treating the emulsified brain with formalin. Dr. Neal states: "The results have been variable, on the whole somewhat encouraging."

Gay rendered rabbits immune by intracerebral injection of a dermotropic strain of herpes virus. He used the brains of rabbits found to be immune to make a vaccine which he calls hyperimmune rabbit vaccine. Another vaccine, also prepared by Gay and Holden, consisted of a formalized herpes virus. Both vaccines have been given in weekly intervals, three doses of 2 cc. each and fifteen doses of 4 cc. each.

Neal has compared the results obtained from all the vaccines mentioned. She believes that an evaluation of improvement is difficult because the natural course of the disease is irregular. The best results were obtained with Gay's hyperimmune rabbit brain vaccine and Levaditi's vaccine (48 per cent improved out of 350 cases). Rosenow's vaccine she considers to be only a nonspecific protein without marked effect. Good results have been obtained in a small group of patients treated with the new formalized virus vaccine, but, says Neal, "the value of the vaccine has not yet definitely been proven."

In summary, one must admit that the results obtained from treatment with various vaccines have not been too encouraging. I believe that vaccines are only a form of nonspecific protein therapy, for, were it specific, one could reasonably expect a higher incidence of favorable results.

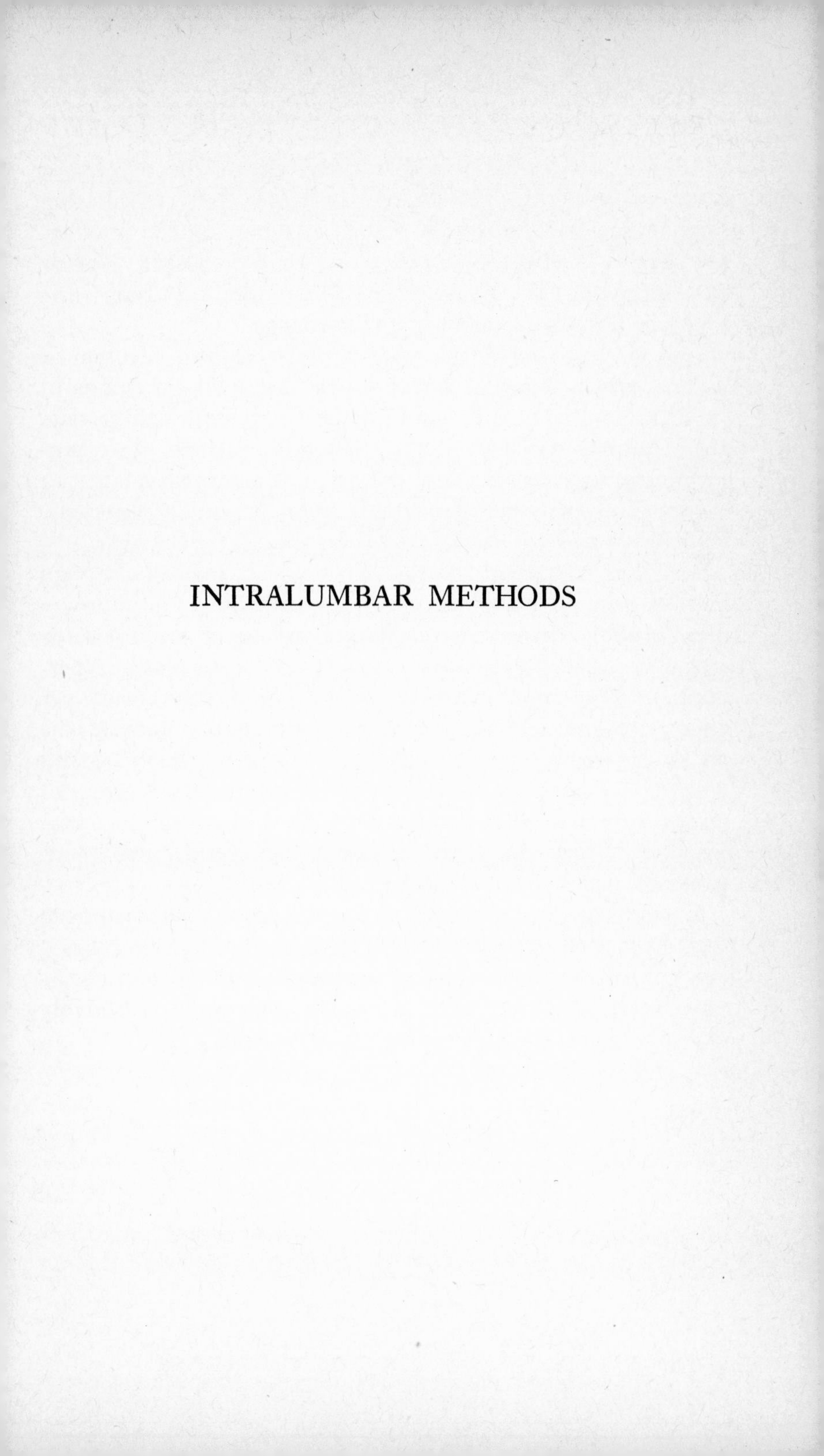

INTRALUMBAR METHODS

Chapter 6

INTRALUMBAR METHODS

The intrathecal method has been employed in an attempt to bring medication closer to the brain. Whether this is possible or whether a uniform admixture of medicine and spinal fluid can occur is seriously open to question, primarily because of the variability in diffusion. Furthermore, the drug ascends only to the level of the basal cisternae and not to the surface of the brain. Moreover, part of the injected substance is absorbed from the spinal fluid into the blood stream. Thus, for example, iodine is found in the blood fifteen minutes following injection into the spinal canal. All solutions to be injected must be isothermic, since colder solutions produce painful irritations of the cauda and occasionally induce signs of transverse cord section.

Simple lumbar or suboccipital puncture is of value only in cases in which intracranial pressure is high. Patients do not always tolerate the procedure well.

To decrease rigidity, Yoshida performed conventional lumbar anesthesia. Rigidity and cogwheel rigidity disappeared rapidly while voluntary mobility was undisturbed, but tremor disappeared only if voluntary activity disappeared. Proceeding from the well-known fact (Walshe) that novocaine injected into a rigid muscle abolishes the rigidity by paralyzing the afferent fibers, Marinesco, Kreindler and Façon injected 7 cc. of a 1 per cent solution of novocaine intrathecally and ten minutes later observed a marked diminution in the cogwheel rigidity. Though these experiments seem to me to be very interesting, I still find lumbar anesthesia much too dangerous and impractical.

Injecting air into the brain (suboccipitally) is recommended by Benedek and Turzo and also by Medea. After the withdrawal of 20 to 30 cc. of spinal fluid, an equal quantity of air is injected. It is presumed that rigidity is diminished and all movements facilitated. I have not observed good results with this method, but Schuster has described a very interesting case of postencephalitic Parkinsonism with severe character disturbances and attacks of screaming in which this method was apparently successful. The patient became unconscious two to three times daily and during these states shouted uninterruptedly for hours. The spells were accompanied by tonic-clonic seizures and were unaffected by the use of scopolamine. Eighty cc. of fluid were withdrawn and 80 cc. of air injected, after which, the report states, the seizures disappeared permanently.

Marinesco, and Alessandrini and Frattali introduced intrathecal treatment with magnesium sulfate. They injected 0.08 to 1 gram of magnesium sulfate in 10 cc. of water every three days, giving three to four injections. The authors report that the arteriosclerotic rigidity was not influenced, but the Parkinson rigidity and tremor disappeared quickly and permanently.

Stark reports injecting a very dangerous preparation: dihydro-naphtacridine-carbonic acid (tetrophine). He treated nine cases with a 5 per cent solution and got good results.

Roch and Katzenelbogen have made injections of casein, using 0.5 cc. of a 10 per cent solution (0.05 gram casein). Up to 0.4 gram casein were injected. Meningism appeared, but was transient. The authors believe this method to be innocuous to the patient, and that, as the meninges become more permeable, the antibodies increase correspondingly.

In all of my experiments employing intramuscular injections of autogenous whole blood, I have noted little or no effect and have not dared to use the intrathecal route. Naumow, however, did so, using blood mixed with an equal quantity of spinal fluid. He believes that in this manner the subcortical ganglia are stimulated and the biochemical processes in the body are favorably influenced.

In contrast to the intralumbar injection of medicaments, intralumbar serum treatment has produced better results and employs the same rationale—the production of an improved circulation in the region of the brain affected by the disease. Pette has demonstrated by numerous experiments with animals that their own serum, injected into the spinal canal, produced by means of meningeal irritation an enormous increase in the number of cells, especially in the basal meninges at the stem (aseptic meningitis). In the treatment of Parkinsonism, 30 cc. of patient's blood is rendered inactive and 10 cc. of sterile serum is injected. After a few hours, one notes headache, pain in the muscles of the neck, and a rise in temperature to about 38°C. (100°F.), which disappears entirely in six to seven days. The leukocytes are increased up to 4,000 per cubic millimeter but return to normal after eight days. The seriousness of the clinical picture parallels the number of cells in the spinal fluid.

Pette treated twenty-three cases, of whom nine remained uninfluenced while eleven improved, some of them markedly. The first signs of improvement became apparent after about eight days. Speech and motility are improved, but only for a few weeks or months. The reason why some cases respond to treatment and others do not remains obscure. It is possible that in the cases without favorable reaction, the foramina Magendi and Luschka are blocked. Foerster and Klauber have found such blocks on several occasions, while performing pneumoencephalography and Foerster's test with sodium iodine.

Others have also reported good results. Paulian even reports "cured" cases in which rigidity was preponderant, whereas hyperkinesias could not be influenced. He gave the injection once a week, for a total of three to six times. Five cases out of twenty-one were reported to have been completely cured, thirteen improved, while three remained unchanged.

Conti suggests that treatment be instituted as soon as possible after the first appearance of signs of postencephalitic Parkinsonism because, according to him, at the very onset there are many antibodies present. Also Hermann, Moore and Tucker are convinced of the benefits of this treatment. Tucker precedes intrathecal injections by administering 1 cc. hypodermically, in order to test for sensitivity. He has treated nine cases with reportedly remarkable improvement.

Following the theories of Levaditi, vaccine was also given intrathecally. Le Fèvre de Arric treated ten cases, and noted some improvement in two instances. Levaditi, himself, gave an injection of 2 to 4 cc. once weekly up to a total of 6 to 8 cc. and found the results satisfactory in four cases. General symptoms following injection are said to be harmless, but Marie and Poincloux observed meningitic symptoms after the injection of 1 to 5 cc. in a solution of 1:20 once weekly. The same authors and Codet tried another method. They injected 1 cc. and fourteen days later, 2 cc. Temperatures rose to 39.3° C. (102° F), but rapidly returned to normal. A new injection was not followed by a reaction.

Scant importance is ascribed to intralumbar vaccine therapy by reports so far published. The effect is, beyond all doubt, not at all specific but rather nonspecific. Theoretically, intramuscular injection should also produce positive reactions and consequent improvement, but these do not occur. Results of the intralumbar serum treatment are better, especially at the onset of postencephalitic Parkinsonism, but in the present state of our knowledge, it cannot be employed as the sole method of treatment.

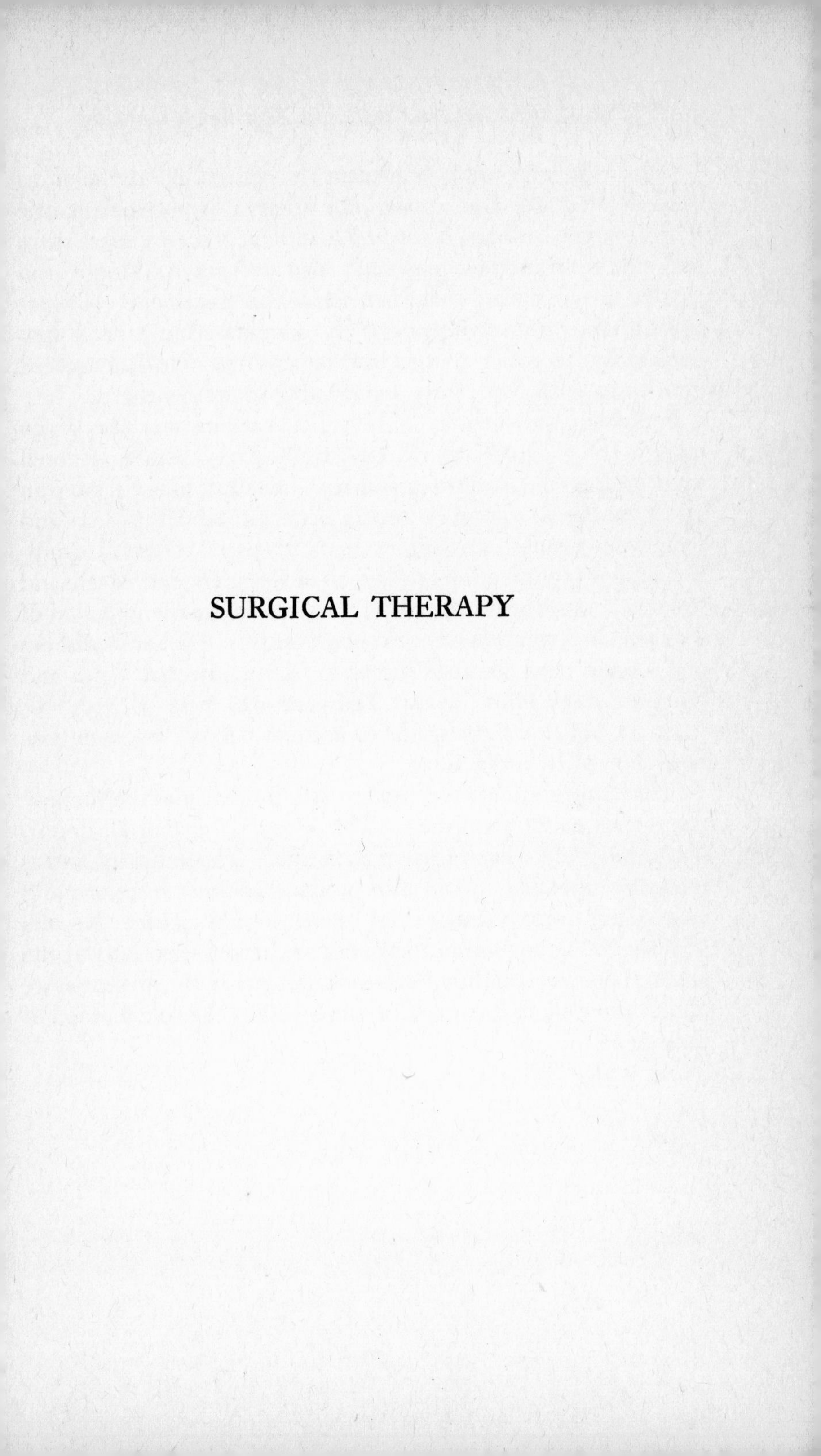

SURGICAL THERAPY

CHAPTER 7

SURGICAL THERAPY

Surgical procedures for the treatment of postencephalitic Parkinsonism have been reported only within relatively recent years, but already great progress can be noted, especially in the United States. One must differentiate between general and special surgical methods. General methods are directed to the amelioration of general symptoms or signs. Special methods are employed to influence the special, unique signs of postencephalitic Parkinsonism and are carried out at the local centers presumably related to these symptoms, i.e., the premotor and motor centers (area 6 and 4), and the pyramidal and extrapyramidal pathways in the spinal cord.

An increased intracranial pressure may occur in chronic relapsing encephalitis and in rare cases of postencephalitic Parkinsonism. Forced drainage, introduced by Kubie in 1926 might be of some value in such cases. As intravenous injection of hypotonic solution and simple trepanation are of transitory value in such cases, incision of the corpus callosum (Balkenstich) has been tried in a few cases with good results. The indications for this operation would seem to be rare. Of 827 cases in my experience none had a sufficient increase in intracranial pressure to warrant such a procedure.

In considering operative intervention, the danger of a general narcosis (ether, chloroform, evipan, avertin) for encephalitics must be borne in mind, since such patients quite often suffer from respiratory disturbances (Jeliffe and others). Grinker and Walker report losing two patients during the operative procedure because of paralysis of the respiratory center.

The use of special surgical treatment of the central nervous system in postencephalitic Parkinsonism was first mentioned by Leriche in 1912, but only during the past ten to fifteen years has definite progress been made, thanks to the work of American and English doctors. Leriche was the first to perform section of the posterior roots, wrongly believing that the rigidity is due to peripheral excitation. As a result, the rigidity remained unchanged, but the tremor diminished. Pollock and Davis were satisfied with the results of the operations. The rigidity of the arm was abolished, but the tremor continued, followed later by contracture. This does not happen after section of posterior roots performed in persons who are not suffering from diseases of the nervous system. The reasons for this are unknown.

The operation performed by Delmas-Marsalet is, as far as I know, original and unique in the entire literature. His thesis is that diseases of the cerebellum are the "negative" of Parkinsonism, and that it should therefore be possible to improve the symptoms of Parkinsonism by producing artificial lesions in the cerebellum. His procedure is to make small burr holes after which he introduces fine needles and applies a current of 10 milliamperes for fifteen minutes. As he anticipated, the rigidity was diminished. The treatment, however, is not without danger, due to the possibility of hemorrhages which, in fact, occurred when this author attempted to produce a lesion in the dentate nucleus as well.

Our present conceptions concerning operative procedures upon the brain and cord in cases of postencephalitic Parkinsonism are founded upon the modern knowledge of the physiology of muscles (Magnus, Foerster, Ken Kuré, and others) and depend upon whether the innervation of the muscles is twofold or threefold. DeBoer has shown that normal muscle tone disappears following section of the sympathetic nerves. Sherrington, Langlaan, and Ken Kuré have demonstrated the sympathetic innervation of striped musculature. On the basis of this proof Royle and Hunter sectioned the rami communicantes grisei in order to diminish the plastic muscle tonus. The rigidity improved slightly, the tremor not at all. Royle treated twenty-two cases of postencephalitic Parkinsonism with the following results:

	cases	*per cent*
Very good improvement	1	4.5
Good improvement	5	22.7
Some improvement	9	40.7
No improvement	7	31.7

Adson, using Royle's technique, had only negative results, whereas Lemoine saw immediate improvement in the rigidity of the legs following section of the lumbar rami communicantes. Section of the second to the fourth lumbar ganglia, in cases of rigidity in the legs, was done transabdominally, a severe procedure in itself. Harrower and Ghosh also observed limited effects after removal of the last cervical and first thoracic ganglia. Kidd, likewise using Royle's technique, removed the superior thoracic ganglion in one patient. The immediate result was: miosis, perspiration of the face on the same side, vasodilatation of the arm, increased temperature, and ptosis. A week later ptosis and vasodilatation disappeared and the patient showed both subjective and objective improvement. Six weeks later the tremor of the arm disappeared. In summarizing the results, it would seem that various sympathectomies performed on postencephalitics have been of doubtful value.

Attempts to improve rigidity and tremor in postencephalitic Parkinsonism by operations on the brain itself arose from the observations of Horsley who for the first time, in 1909, excised the excitable motor cortex (area 6) in a case of athetosis. Involuntary movements were diminished, but voluntary paralysis developed. In the meantime, the importance of area 6 was demonstrated by Arning and Fulton who showed that in primates intention tremor could be abolished by removing the precentral cortex. Bucy and Case reported a case with removal of both areas 4 and 6, following which the tremor disappeared, an improvement not achieved by removal of area 4 alone or by partial destruction of area 6.

Browder and Meyers extirpated the head of the caudate nucleus in two cases of postencephalitic hemiparkinsonism without any side effects. In both cases the tremor disappeared. The clinical improvement was confirmed by electromyography and electroencephalography. The authors state that this operation should be reserved for cases of long duration of the tremor without progression of the clinical picture. These cerebral operations are limited to cases with signs of hemiparkinsonism. Perhaps further experience will yield better results.

Tracy J. Putnam was the first to treat diseases of the extrapyramidal system by operation on the spinal cord. Because operations previously performed, such as section of posterior roots (Leriche, Foerster), and incision of the column of Burdach (Puusepp), were absolutely unsatisfactory, he developed his own concept and technique. At first he performed section of the extrapyramidal tracts in the cord, in a case of postencephalitic Parkinsonism, but without improvement. Since Parkinson, in his first paper (1817), described the disappearance of the tremor if the patient develops an apoplexia, i.e., a lesion of the corticospinal tract, Putnam then tried section of the pyramidal tract. In several cases he noted good results with regard to the tremor, which vanished or was reduced to "an insignificant remnant." All the cases improved, but Putnam is properly cautious in his conclusions. "Whether any of these operations can be used in bilateral cases is open to question. The entire question is a new one."

Other operations are performed to improve other signs of postencephalitic Parkinsonism. In cases with oculogyric crises, for example, Grafar and Spitzmuller electrocoagulated the nerve fibers of the eyelid which innervate the muscles closing the eye.

A peculiar operation is described by Myerson and Berliner. They state that in untreated cases of postencephalitic Parkinsonism the metabolism is increased from 15 to 60 per cent in severe cases, dropping when alkaloids are administered. It seemed to them that the normal activity of the thyroid is too great in these cases. On this basis, the thyroid was totally removed and the patient became myxedematous. The authors hoped that the symptoms would be ameliorated after the myxedema was controlled by thyroid extract. Unfortunately, the practical result of this theory was poor. The patient became more tremulous and had to have $\frac{1}{50}$ gram of hyoscine twice daily together with $\frac{1}{2}$ to $\frac{3}{4}$ gram of thyroid. The logical conclusion that there is no foundation for this theory becomes apparent.

Surgical methods are applicable for the treatment of torticollis spastica in postencephalitic Parkinsonism. Section of the accessorius nerve is an ineffectual procedure because the spasm migrates to neighboring groups of muscles or to the other side. Kocher recommends bilateral section of the spastic neck muscles, but these muscles grow together very soon after the operation. A difficult but occasionally successful operation is the extravertebral section of the first three cervical nerves (Keen, Finney, and Hughson). A less difficult procedure is the bilateral intradural section of the first three upper anterior and posterior roots, together with section of the accessorius nerve of the affected side. Dandy has cut only the motor roots, reporting good results.

As mentioned previously, encephalitics often suffer from disturbances in respiration. In cases with a tic of the diaphragm Gamble and others exposed the phrenic nerves bilaterally and froze them with chlorethyl, with immediate success. Following radical section of both phrenic nerves by Skillern, the tic disappeared, but returned nine months later. Bilateral exeresis was thereupon performed and the tic disappeared permanently.

Orthopedic operations are seldom performed. Experienced

orthopedists, including Lange and Spitzer, are becoming increasingly reserved and will not operate unless all conservative methods have been previously attempted. In my experience, I have not yet been compelled to refer any cases of postencephalitic Parkinsonism for orthopedic suggestions or surgery.

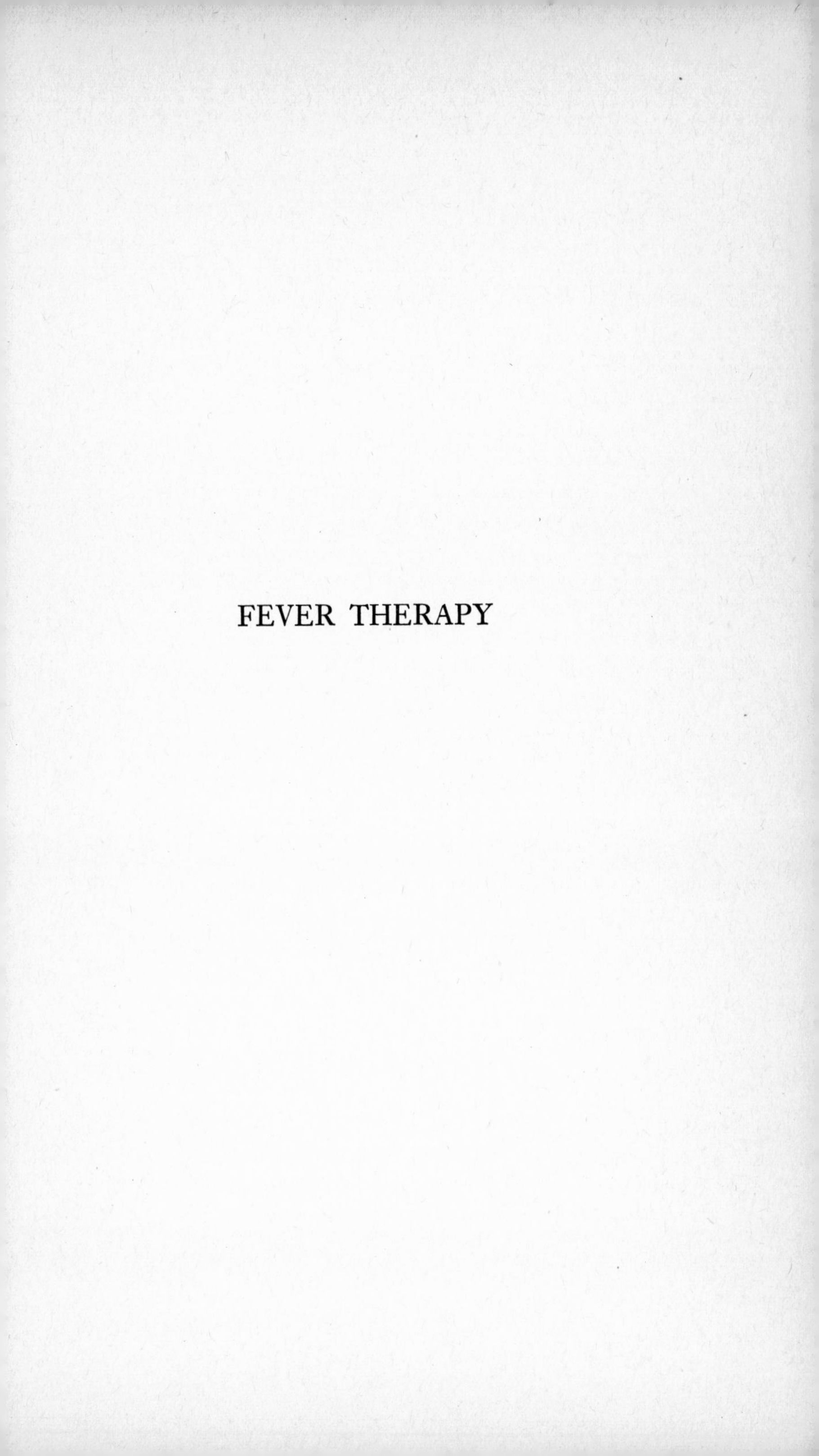

FEVER THERAPY

Chapter 8

FEVER THERAPY

During the last twenty years, fever therapy has been used not only in the treatment of general paresis, but also of several other diseases of the central nervous system. It is therefore not surprising that it has also been tried in postencephalitic Parkinsonism. Regardless of the sort of fever therapy selected for use, one rule must never be overlooked, namely, that so long as a patient is under the influence of alkaloids such as atropine, hyoscine, or Bulgakur, he should never be given any kind of fever treatment. These alkaloids have a direct influence on the temperature regulating center, which makes the combination of fever therapy and alkaloids a very dangerous one. Alkaloids must therefore be curtailed prior to the inception of fever therapy.

The manner in which fever operates upon the brain is not yet known. It is possible that fever strengthens the defense mechanisms of the body. The technique of inducing fever by malaria is similar to that employed in general paresis, and it is important that during the treatment patients be carefully supervised by specially trained personnel.

Embden in Hamburg was the first (1926) to recommend treatment of postencephalitic Parkinsonism by malaria, though Lust had previously published a paper (1921) on postencephalitic sleep disturbances in children which he had successfully treated with artificial fever. Embden believed that fever therapy had a favorable influence on inflammatory processes. The duration of the illness seems to bear some relation to the results of the treatment. At times it is difficult to produce fever in patients with postencephalitic Parkinsonism, and it has been necessary to re-inoculate some of them as often as three times.

A poor state of the general physical condition, old age, and cardiovascular diseases constitute contraindications. According to Embden, Parkinsonians tolerate the treatment better than paretics, an opinion with which I am unable to agree, since in my experience, which is confirmed by that of Stern, and McCowan and Cook, the former are very sensitive, become exhausted and recover very slowly from each attack. I have seen several instances of fatal bronchopneumonia occurring during recovery.

So far as I know, only Stefani has reported spontaneous injection with malaria in postencephalitic Parkinsonism, and in his case the patient's Parkinsonian symptoms and signs promptly became worse. Some authors, among them Craig and McCowan and Cook, prefer natural infection by Anopheles rather than the inoculation method. I myself tried the malaria treatment early in 1927, although Wagner von Jauregg had warned against its use, but after having adverse and fatal results, I abandoned the method very soon and have not tried it since. Table 3 summarizes the experience of several authors. Others not mentioned in the Table also had results which were not at all encouraging.

RECURRENT FEVER THERAPY (TREPONEMA DUTTONI)

Only a few have employed this form of fever therapy in postencephalitic Parkinsonism. Stern as well as Bifulco and Ebhardt achieved very little with it, whereas Kling and Höglund (1926) were satisfied with their results, as were Höglund and Sjögren. A total of forty-one cases were treated, twenty-five of which were grave, with a course of three to six paroxysms. In 61 per cent improvement was said to be obvious, especially in regard to the akinesia. The hyperkinesia, however, was unchanged. The authors found that the duration of the disease bears directly upon the results of treatment; the shorter the Parkinsonism the better are the results. The blood smear is of importance and must be closely observed During the attack there is a leukocytosis with an eosinophilia. After the attack and during the intervals leukopenia, relative lymphocytosis and monocytosis are found. Simultaneously, there is a thrombopenia and an increase in the blood sedimentation rate. Höglund and Sjögren state that all untreated cases became progressively worse, whereas the treated patients were sufficiently improved to resume work. The disease showed an obvious tendency towards remission. The mortality in untreated cases was eight out of thirty-one, in treated cases, three out of fifty-two.

Treponema hispanicum was employed by Mas de Ayala. The fever attack persisted for four days, followed by an afebrile

TABLE 3

Results of malaria treatment

AUTHOR	NUMBER OF CASES	RECOVERED	MARKEDLY IMPROVED	SLIGHTLY IMPROVED	NOT IMPROVED	DEATH
Bohne	3				3	
Craig	8			8		
Gillespie	18	1	4	7	4	2
Herschmann	32		5	3	24	
Kürbitz	12			1	11	
McCowan and Cook	15				15	
von Witzleben	12				9	3
Total	100	1	9	19	66	5

interval of three to five days. This cycle was repeated three times. The patients felt poorly, complaining of severe headaches, vomiting and spells of excessive perspiration. In the event that treponemas are still found in the blood after the fourth paroxysm, 0.3 gram of salvarsan is administered. The author treated eleven cases and observed quick and adequate improvement, especially in relatively recent cases.

ARTIFICIAL FEVER

In producing artificial fever, a great number of preparations have been employed. In the treatment of Parkinsonism, fever induced by typhoid vaccine (Hoff, Renaud), and sterile milk proved to be complete failures. The opinions with regard to sulphur preparations are quite diverse. K. Schroeder finds sulfosin, his own preparation, satisfactory, noting marked improvement in five cases. Stiefler, also employing sulfosin, observed only partial improvement in fifteen cases. Rosenthal gave sulfogel every four to six days, increasing the doses from 0.2 to 6.0 cc., with the resulting fever up to 40°C. (104°F.), but had no success. Adam used a solution of the following composition:

	grams
Sulph. dep.	1.0
Ol. Oliv.	80.0
Eucalyptol	20.0

1 cc. (0.01 gram sulphate) is given as the first injection, intramuscularly, in severe cases 0.5 cc. every four to six days. The dose is increased by 1 cc. up to the maximal dose of 6 to 7 cc. to a total of ten to twelve injections. If the patient complains of severe pain and is in poor physical condition, the next dose should not be increased. Five cases out of nine improved both objectively and subjectively, including the faculties of speaking and swallowing, and improvement lasted for several months. Saprovitan (Dreyfus and Hanau) as well as pyrifer were tried without success. Both are nonspecific protein bodies.

Treatment with fever produced by hot baths or electricity was first applied in luetic diseases of the central nervous system, but is now also administered to patients suffering from postencephalitic Parkinsonism. Developed in 1927 by Wielinski and others, the method made rapid progress, especially in America (C. A. Neymann). The treatment with hot baths introduced by Mehrtens and Pouppirt is only of historical interest today, the electrical bath now in use being more practical and less dangerous. The improvement noted was only subjective. Neymann observed fatal results, whereas treatment with electropyrexia is harmless, if applied properly. The patient must be closely observed by a physician and the personnel must be specially trained. The modern air-conditioned cabinets devised by Simpson, Kislig and Sittler, and Neymann and Holmquest are especially advantageous. It does not seem advisable for the general practitioner to give this treatment, as special and prolonged experience with it is necessary. Treatment is best given in a special department of a hospital, where a skilled personnel and special physicians are available. Extreme caution is called for in cases of heart diseases. Neymann states that cases with rheumatic conditions may be treated. A decompensated heart, however, as well as kidney diseases and severe cerebral arteriosclerosis are absolute contraindications. Patients with syringomyelia, or other diseases producing anesthesia of the body surfaces, should obviously not be given fever treatment. Marasmus and pregnancy are contraindications, but Neymann is said to have successfully treated a pregnant woman. This author feels that the results in postencephalitic Parkinsonism have been quite satisfactory and he feels "that the progress of the disease is delayed or may even be checked after twenty treatments with electropyrexia." The tremor, the rigidity, and the oculogyric crises are diminished. By improving the blood circulation, more antibodies may be brought to the brain. Neymann treats his cases twice weekly, increasing the temperature up to 105°F. for eight hours and giving a total of twenty treatments in all. It is interesting that this treatment is without result in cases of true paralysis agitans.

In summarizing the results of fever treatment, one finds that they have not been very encouraging up to the present. Neither malaria nor artificial fever have produced substantially consistent results, and in addition there have been, on occassion, dangerous consequences. Perhaps electropyrexia may prove to be more successful, but one must wait for further reports as to results. So far the total number of cases treated with electropyrexia and subsequently reported has been too small to warrant the drawing of conclusions.

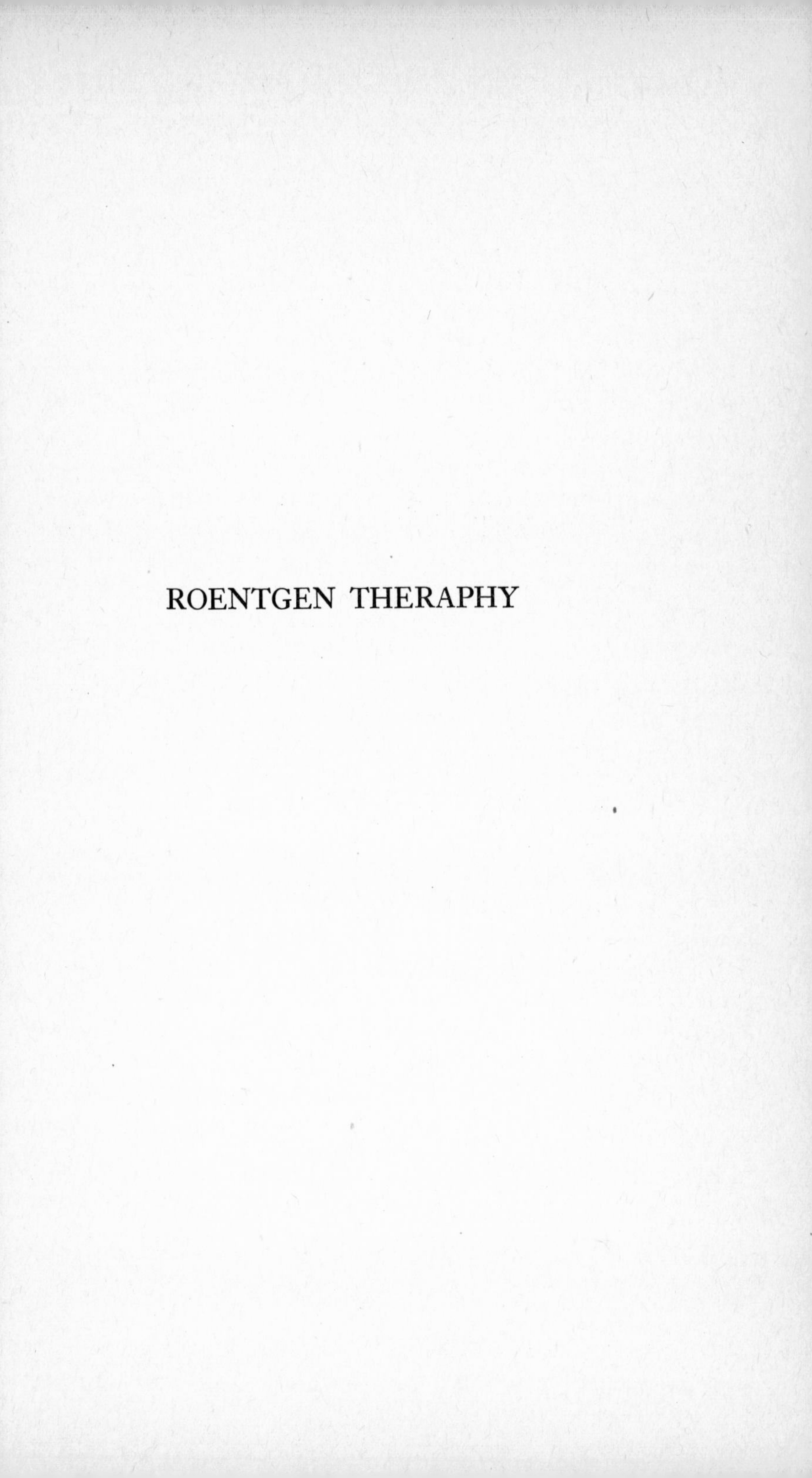

ROENTGEN THERAPHY

Chapter 9

ROENTGEN THERAPY

Effective treatment of organic diseases of the central nervous system by roentgen rays has been reported by Marburg and Sgalitzer, by myself, and by others. X-rays seem to exert an ameliorating affect upon inflammations of various tissues, so that their use to relieve inflammatory diseases of the brain is therapeutically possible, though the brain tissue itself is very resistant to X-rays, and microscopic lesions are found only after irradiation with doses so high that they are well beyond practical therapeutic use.

The fact that Parkinsonian patients have an unusual skin sensitivity, a factor which I have pointed out in previous reports and which Appelrath and others have verified, assumes special importance in superficial irradiation of the parotid gland as a means of diminishing excessive salivation. This latter method was first employed by M. Fraenkel, who noticed, during the last World War, that wounds of the face adjacent to the parotid gland healed poorly because of excessive salivation. The method employed is to administer $\frac{3}{4}$ H.E.D. (*Haut-Einheits-Dosis*—unit skin dose) through 4 millimeters of aluminum. In a few hours an erythema appears, which after a period of four to six weeks assumes a deep brown coloration. By this method one avoids destruction of the gland, while its secretion becomes diminished or is temporarily eliminated.

For irradiation of the skull, the technique employed by the Viennese radiologist, von Wieser, is often used. This method is as follows: 180 to 200 K.V. under 0.5 millimeter zinc and 1 millimeter aluminum. The areas of exposure on the skull are 6 to 8 centimeters in diameter, on the vertebral column 6 centimeters in width and long enough to divide the spinal cord into approximate thirds. In milder cases the focal skin distance should be 30 centimeters, in more severe cases 50 centimeters. In severe cases one area is exposed during one period, employing 5 to 10 per cent H.E.D. (30 to 60 R.), in mild cases two areas in one period, with 25 to 30 per cent H.E.D. (150 to 200 R.) The areas of the skull are distributed as follows: one longitudinal area each, on left (L) and right (R) temple, the base of this area so placed that the antrum of Highmore is also irradiated; frontally (F) the area reaches as far as the anterior fossa of the skull; one proximal area of the forehead, so placed that the central ray runs parallel to the base of the skull and the lower margin of the area is about 1 centimeter below the base of the skull.

On the spinal cord the areas exposed are: 1) occiput and cervical vertebral column (O.C.V.); 2) superior and median thoracic vertebral column (T.V.); 3) inferior thoracic vertebral column and lumbar vertebral column (L.V.).

One series consists of six to twelve irradiations. Alternating irradiations of cranial and dorsal areas respectively are given, for example: R—O.C.V; L—T.V; F—L.V. This course may be given twice in succession. In mild cases, exposures are made once a month over two areas (25 to 30 per cent H.E.D. for each area); in more severe cases, one or two exposures a week to one area each (10 per cent H.E.D. per area). In mild cases an interval of four weeks after each two irradiations is allowed; while in more severe cases a four-week interval is allowed after the first series of twelve irradiations, six weeks after the second, eight weeks after the third, and twelve weeks after the fourth series. In cases with postencephalitic Parkinsonism, a pause should be made after eight to ten weeks of irradiation for a rest period of two to three months. If the doses are too large and the rest intervals too brief, a relapse may occur after an initial success. The dose employed should be governed not only by the general condition of the patient, but also by the course and progress of the disease. If the illness progresses rapidly, smaller doses should be employed and the rest intervals more freely spaced.

Little is to be found in the literature concerning the results of X-ray treatment in postencephalitic Parkinsonism. The results of my own experience with roentgen treatment have been far from gratifying. Goldberg too reports poor results. He employed intermediate doses of 135 K.V., 5 milliamperes, at a distance of 38 centimeters, under 3 millimeters aluminum, 40 r. One series consisted of ten to twelve exposures. P. Krause, an experienced and critical physician, has succeeded in ameliorating the symptoms in seven out of thirteen cases, four rather remarkably. The rigidity decreased and muscular movements became easier within a period varying from eleven days up to six weeks after treatment. He used 180 K.V., 4 milliamperes at a distance of 30 centimeters, under 0.5 millimeter copper and 1 millimeter aluminum, on four skull and one neck areas, 10 to 15 per cent H.E.D. daily. A second series was applied after three months.

Pansdorf and Trautmann believe that irradiation increases the bactericidal power of the blood serum and destroys lymphocytes and leukocytes in the area of the inflammation. Their technique, after the Holfelder scheme, is: 200 K.V., 7 milliamperes, 0.5 millimeter copper, at a distance of 40 centimeters 10–15–20 per cent H.E.D., repeated after four to eight days, for a total of three exposures. They did not succeed, however, in improving any case of postencephalitic Parkinsonism.

Vor der Brück has practised this technique in all of his cases of postencephalitic Parkinsonism since 1933, believing that the treatment produces an improved blood circulation in the basal ganglia and facilitates discharge of the inflammatory infiltrations. The doses he employs are quite high and are intended to stimulate the atrophic ganglion cells. His technique is: 170 K.V., 6 milliamperes, 40 centimeters distance, through 1.0 millimeter copper and 1.0 millimeter aluminum, 40 to 60 per cent H.E.D. (240 to 360 R.), five areas, each 6 to 8 centimeters, every two to three days. He administers 50 per cent dextrose intravenously for complaints following the irradiation. The series is repeated after three to four months. In some cases, the objective and subjective disturbances were accentuated shortly after treatment began and remained so for about six weeks. In all, only ten cases were treated, of which seven showed slight improvement, lasting no longer than six months, after which the disease became progressive.

A somewhat different technique is described by Kiss and Szirmak. In accordance with the observations made by both Royle and Hunter that sections of the brain below the red nucleus did not produce rigidity if the superior thoracic ganglia of the opposite side were removed, Kiss and Szirmak irradiated the medial cervical and superior thoracic ganglion (spinal cord 10 centimeters down the vertebra prominens, 10 centimeters large, perpendicular to the mid-line of the spinal column). Rather marked reactions, lasting four to five days, appear, particularly an increase in tremor and speech disturbances, and are then followed by a decrease in salivation, tremors and rigidity. A relapse can be quickly aborted with another treatment. It is noteworthy that no true paralysis agitans reacted favorably. Untoward sequelae have not occurred, but children are sometimes unusually sensitive and may become sleepy (Druckmann) or, as reported by Lorey and Schaltenbrand, may develop pachymeningitis.

Judging from the results, which have not been sufficiently gratifying, it seems to me that X-ray treatment should not be administered to adult patients with postencephalitic Parkinsonism. On the other hand, it may be tried for character disturbances and in treating erethistic adolescents, because of the quieting action of irradiation, which von Wieser and others have noted as resulting from such treatment of these patients.

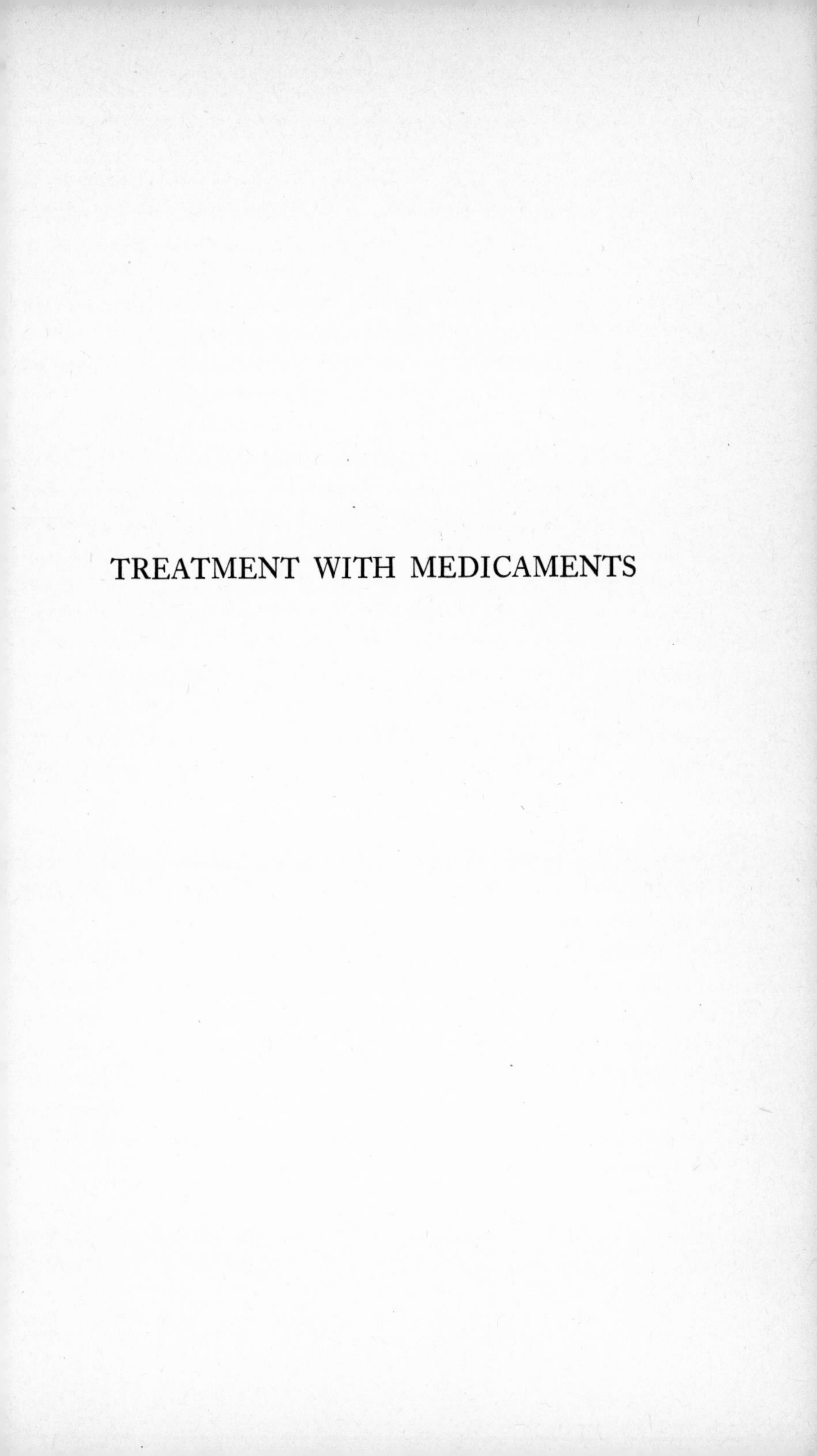

TREATMENT WITH MEDICAMENTS

Chapter 10

TREATMENT WITH MEDICAMENTS

Sedatives, hypnotics and analgesics do not influence the signs of postencephalitic Parkinsonism directly. Though they are often administered because of various subjective complaints, it is my conviction that one should avoid use of these drugs as much as possible.

Almost all of the sedatives used in Parkinsonism belong to the group of barbituric acid derivatives. Cooper gives bromide and luminal to decrease the oculogyric crises. Leak reports satisfying results from the administration of ½ tablet of prominal in the morning, for oculogyric crises. Luminal, prominal or bromide are given for epileptic seizures. Paraldehyde may be used for periods of excitement, but there are certain disadvantages in the use of any of the barbiturates, and they are sometimes dangerous (Runge, Ziskind and Sommerfeld-Ziskind). Even in cases of sleep disturbances they are without effect. Phenobarbital has a direct influence on the brain stem, and Claude and Baruk believe that it should not be used in postencephalitic Parkinsonism because the connections between the cortex and brain stem are disturbed. Stern also points out that the barbiturates cannot act as a sedative for a destroyed area.

Frensdorf has noted hallucinations after the use of phenobarbital. Moreover, it is well known that chronic use of veronal in large quantities produces a Parkinson-like picture, with rigidity and hallucinations. Ziskind and Sommerfeld-Ziskind report a severe aggravation in a patient who by error took 0.1 gram phenobarbital three times a day for four days, instead of his usual doses of scopolamine.

Judging from my own experience, these warnings seem to be completely justified. In my opinion, barbiturates should not be used, except in cases of epilepsy, whether or not the seizures are due to chronic encephalitis. As will be shown further on, the oculogyric crises can be influenced by other and more efficacious means.

Duensing and Meyer recommend intravenous injections of calcibronat. In many cases I have had occasion to notice that similar results can be obtained by injections of water or saline solutions, as Parkinsonian patients are very amenable to any sort of suggestion.

Morphine should never be given.

Analgesics can be given to patients with neurotic pains, rheumatism, and so on. If the pain is unusually severe and cannot be controlled by irradiation, as for example, in cases with a thalamic syndrome, cobra venom may be helpful. The average dose is 5 mouse units, intramuscularly, one mouse unit being the quantity of cobra venom fatal within eighteen hours after intraperitoneal injection into a mouse weighing twenty-four grams (Gayle and Williams). The first day 0.5 cc. is given, the second, 1 cc., up to a total of ten injections

All attempts at treatment with glandular preparations, such as implantation of parathyroids or intravenous injection of 0.02 gram parathyroids three times a day for two to three months, have failed to produce any significant results. On the other hand, ephedrine and benzedrine are very effective when indicated. For example, ephedrine is helpful in all cases of narcolepsy. Sleep disturbances are prominent in many cases of postencephalitic Parkinsonism; such patients are often sleepless or show the conversion type of sleep, sleeping during the day and being awake at night. I have found ephedrine very helpful in all such cases, only a small dose ($\frac{1}{4}$ to $\frac{1}{2}$ tablet) being necessary, to be given not later than noon. A patient, described in a previous report of mine, was tired and sleepy all day, frequently fell asleep during working hours and faced discharge from work. Ephedrine ($\frac{1}{4}$ to $\frac{1}{2}$ tablet) given at 7 a.m. was sufficient to counteract the sleepiness during the day, without effecting the normal sleep at night. The patient was able to carry on his work and had no further complaints of sleep disturbance.

Benzedrine has also been found useful in postencephalitic Parkinsonism. As can be seen from its formula, benzedrine (amphetamine sulfate) is closely related to ephedrine.

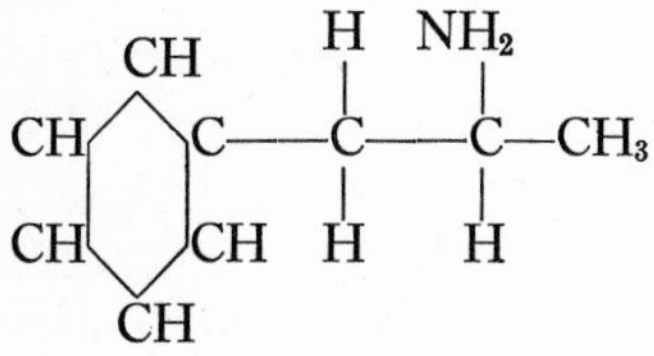

```
        CH     H  NH2          |           OH      OH NHCH3
                |   |          |                    |     |
 CH/  \C----C----C--CH3        |   CH/  \C-----C--------C--CH3
   |    |       |   |          |     |    |    |        |
 CH\  /CH   H   H              |   CH\  /CH    H        H
        CH                     |          CH
      Benzedrine               |          Epinephrine
```

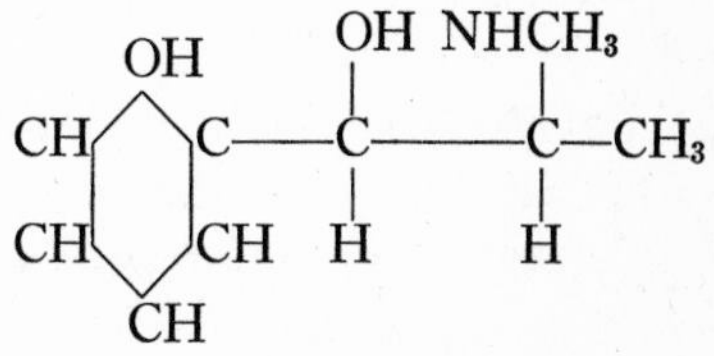

Since 1930, pharmacological experiments with benzedrine have been performed on animals and in 1935 Prinzmetal and Bloomberg made the first therapeutic trials on patients suffering from narcolepsy.

Benzedrine is a sympathicomimetic remedy with a central and peripheral action. Given in small doses, it renders the patient euphoric and somewhat hyperactive. There may be some side effects such as perspiration, tachycardia, arrhythmia, anxiety, nausea, vomiting and insomnia. Blood counts should be done, since Davis and Stewart have, in rare cases, noted the occurrence of aplastic anemia. Heart diseases, especially when there is increased blood pressure and diseased coronary arteries, are contraindications to its use. Benzedrine, like all amines of the type of $R.CH_2NH_2$, is quickly eliminated, although Myerson and others state that it is not rapidly destroyed in the tissues and remains for quite a long time in the blood stream.

In cases of postencephalitic Parkinsonism with true depression, great caution should be exercised in the use of benzedrine. As mentioned above, patients are apt to become euphoric under the influence of benzedrine, while at the same time there is a cessation of inhibition. In this state patients are extremely suicidal.

The proper dose must be individually calibrated, beginning with small amounts, for example 2½ milligrams each before breakfast and lunch. Since benzedrine interferes with sleep, it should not be given in the afternoon and evening. The effect appears from one-half to one hour after the drug is taken and may last three, six, or seventeen hours. The dose should be increased slowly by 2½ milligrams each, until the smallest optimal effective dose is found.

The results of benzedrine treatment in postencephalitic Parkinsonism have not been uniform. In my own experience there have been no satisfactory results when benzedrine alone was used, nor did I find it superior to alkaloids. It has, however, an objectively salutary influence on the mood and on the oculogyric crises.

Reznikoff, Davidoff, and others have shown that it is fundamentally impossible to change the structure of a psychosis, so that in cases with real psychoses, benzedrine has no effect whatsoever. Reznikoff tried 10 milligrams twice daily, to a total of 2,200 milligrams. Euphoria was obvious, but when the medication was stopped, the patient soon relapsed to his former state. As little as 20 milligrams of benzedrine may produce severe states of rage and excitement in some patients, while others are known to tolerate as much as 160 milligrams daily without any untoward disturbances.

According to Gargant and Blackburn, the intelligence score increases by approximately 8 per cent after the use of benzedrine. Here, however, one is not dealing with an absolute increase, the effect being caused by the improvement in mood. The effect of benzedrine may be enhanced by combining it with atropine (Finkelman and Shapiro) or scopolamine and stramonium (Fressler; Matthews; Solomon, Mitchell and Prinzmetal). Also, the combination with alkaloids (belladonna) may bring some benefit in a few cases.

I agree with other workers in this field that the beneficial effect of benzedrine is principally upon oculogyric crises and psychic abnormalities with the exception of the severe psychoses. In such cases, good results can be obtained if benzedrine is combined with alkaloids. Adult behavior and character disorders should not, in my opinion, be treated with benzedrine, since these patients are inclined per se to excitement, impulsive actions, and so on.

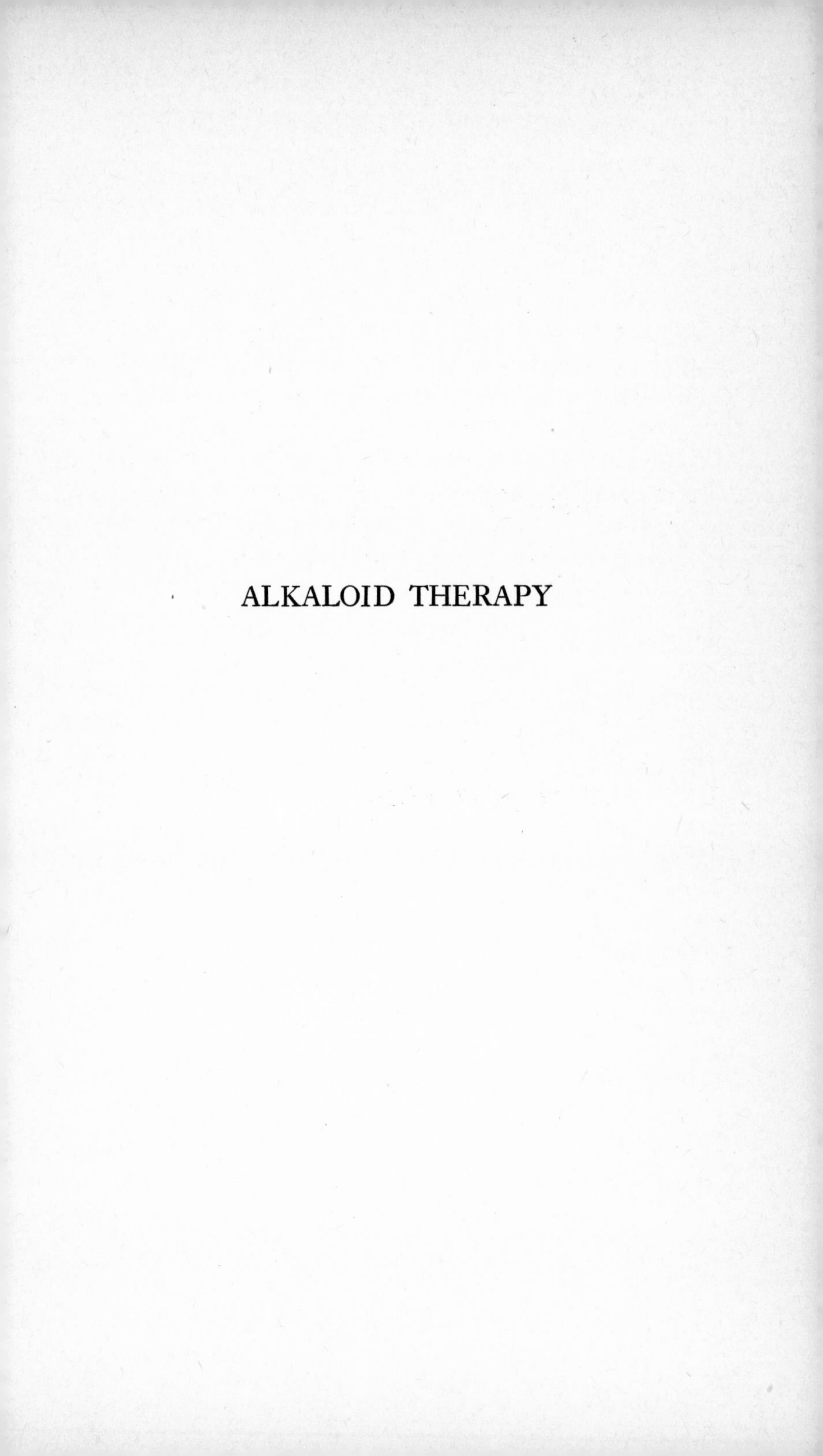

ALKALOID THERAPY

CHAPTER II

ALKALOID THERAPY

Some of the foregoing methods of treatment have a substantial degree of usefulness when the symptoms are simple, but are less useful when the full picture of postencephalitic Parkinsonism is considered. Their respective effects, however, have been surpassed by the use of alkaloid therapy, as it has developed within the past fifteen years, which now, in turn, has been supplanted by the Bulgarian treatment.

NICOTINE

Comparatively speaking, minimal effects have been noted with the use of three other alkaloids: nicotine, curare, and bulbocapnine. As suggested in Chapter 2, the use of tobacco is discouraged whenever possible, since nicotine apparently aggravates the state of many patients. It is surprising, therefore, and not yet entirely clear that Hermann and Wotke successfully treated with nicotine a patient with postencephalitic Parkinsonism, who had told them that his tremor was much improved after having smoked quite heavily. They administered 1 to 2 milligrams of nicotinum tartaricum, without success. More effective was a decoction of cigarette tobacco, using a dose of 0.59 milligrams of dry substance. Favorable effects in two cases lasted eight and twenty days respectively. The other cases showed some improvement, but only for a few hours. Contrary to the usual effect of nicotine, these patients showed a great desire for sleep.

Noll noted improvement in nine out of thirteen cases. The shortening and lengthening reaction was diminished, using $\frac{1}{30}$ grain three times a day and increasing the dose up to $\frac{1}{10}$ or

$\frac{1}{5}$ grain. No effect upon the tremor could be noted, but—in contradistinction to Herrmann and Wotke's observations—the rigidity was somewhat improved. One cannot, of course, arrive at any definite conclusions from these statements; in the light of my own experiences, I still believe that nicotine not only does little substantial good, but can actually be harmful.

CURARE

Curare, the mysterious arrow poison of the Indians, has been used repeatedly in the treatment of postencephalitic Parkinsonism. Its physiological action was first studied and described by Claude Bernard in 1846, and in 1869 Jousset, Dermmic and Busch treated chorea, rabies, and epilepsy with this drug. Bernard believed the effect to be produced by a block of the nervous impulses at the myoneural junctions (motor end-plate), so that acetylcholine, which normally acts at this point, is inhibited from doing so. In the use of curare, one must watch for side effects, such as drop in blood pressure, erythema, and other histamine-like reactions, which can be relieved by ephedrine or epinephrine.

West successfully treated twenty cases showing spasm and rigidity, both of which diminished following injections of 2 to 20 milligrams of the drug.

Curare is administered intramuscularly or intravenously, beginning with a small dose and gradually increasing it until the individually effective dose is reached. This is the maximum to be injected at one time. The first effects appear about twenty to thirty minutes following intramuscular injection, while after intravenous injection they appear immediately. The patient feels dizzy and it becomes difficult for him to raise his eyelids, as in myasthenia gravis. According to Burman, it is impossible to produce complete flaccidity in an extremity (within the therapeutic range), but the muscular rigidity is released and the muscles become much looser.

Such complicated movements as holding a glass of water, and the like, also become possible. Apparently, there are some variations in the sensitivity of certain muscle groups to curare; thus, a soft rigidity responds better than a fixed one, while palmar flexion of the wrist is extremely difficult to influence. It is therefore wiser to abstain from treating fixed deformities.

It is noteworthy that curare has an effect upon torticollis and torsion dystonia (dystonia musculorum deformans), such patients tolerating surprisingly large doses—25 milligrams intravenously. The salutary effects remain for several days. The improvement is slight, however, when the dystonia is combined with extreme rigidity.

Unfortunately, curare is not easy to obtain. Burman, Bennett, and others therefore tried erythroidine, which, according to the U.S.P. is "a powerful motor paralysant." Altamirano isolated the drug out of Erythrina coralloides in 1888. It is injected intravenously in the form of erythroidine hydrochloride (300 to 950 milligrams). The therapeutic effect is not as good as that of curare, and it causes more undesirable side effects, such as diplopia, slight nystagmus, and palsy of the upper lid. When given perorally, it is without effect, even when the dose is as high as 3,000 milligrams.

Kairiukschtis and Kutorga have given 1.5 to 2 cc. of kuraril, a 0.5 per cent solution of curare, intravenously. The rigidity improved slightly, while tremor and salivation remained unchanged.

In view of the results now established, it seems doubtful whether the use of curare is to be recommended. It should be stressed that certain side effects resulting from its use may be quite harmful.

BULBOCAPNINE

In its chemical composition bulbocapnine is closely allied to apomorphine, except that it is optically dextrorotary, while apomorphine is levorotary.

Gadamar developed the following formula:

H
H OCH_3
OH
H_2
H
CH_3N O
CH_2
H_2 O
H_2 H

The drug is administered hypodermically or perorally, and is for the most part eliminated from the kidneys in an unaltered form. The side effects noted are a fall in blood pressure, slow respiration, fatigue, dizziness, and retardation of mental activity. The mechanism by which the drug operates is not yet well known. In 1904, Peters described cataleptic-like phenomena involving the voluntary and reflex movements, whereas proprioception and tonus of the musculature remained unchanged. Schaltenbrand studied bulbocapnine poisoning in dogs, apes, and men, and noted that if 0.01 gram per kilogram of body weight is administered to man a feeling of fatigue results. With larger doses, all psychic activities become retarded, and a feeling of approaching narcosis is experienced.

DeJong states that bulbocapnine catalepsy is not a true catalepsy. In the poisoned animal, one cannot bring an extremity into a desired position and keep it so, as it always returns to the resting position. Froehlich and Meyer state that in bulbocapnine poisoning there is no action current, but intermittent action currents can be recorded with the galvanometer of Wertheim-Solomonson. Bulbocapnine does not produce a tonic contraction—since it does not disappear following application of novocaine—but rather a tetanic contracture on which novocaine is without influence.

Sensitivity to bulbocapnine can be enhanced by lesions of

the brain, for example, in the region of the red nucleus. When the retromammilary region is injured, catalepsy appears and the animals become exquisitely sensitive to small doses of bulbocapnine. These experiments suggest that, in similar manner, it might be possible to influence some of the symptoms of postencephalitic Parkinsonism. When the drug is taken orally, patients often complain of stomach trouble, and it becomes necessary to add sodium bicarbonate to the bulbocapnine, viz.,

℞		
℞	Bulbocapnine hydrochloride	1.0
	Sodium bicarbonate	0.1
	Acidum tartaricum	0.1
	Saccharum lacticum	0.8
	Saccharini	0.01
	M. F. tabl. X	

Pills must be covered with stearic acid which guarantees that the drug is dissolved only in the intestine.

When given parenterally, it is preferable to combine bulbocapnine hydrochloride or phosphorus with olive oil or gum arabicum, thereby creating a depot for the purpose of slow, uniform absorption. While 0.2 milligram bulbocapnine is effective for about three hours, as little as 0.15 milligram bulbocapnine in gum arabicum is active for almost seven hours. Sublingual administration diminishes or causes the disappearance of the tremor for one day, but pills for two and one-half hours only. This medication may be given without danger for months, and there will be no signs of deprivation if it is suddenly stopped. Leiner and Kaufman treated eight cases using 0.1–0.2 milligram hypodermically, and observed beneficial but irregular effects on the tremor although the muscular hypertony remained unchanged.

Levy, Fleischhacker and others have not observed any beneficial results from the administration of bulbocapnine. In addition, it is expensive and difficult to obtain; its use, therefore, cannot be recommended at the present time. On the other hand, Clerici, Hill, and Jenkins and Rowley seem quite content with the results obtained in cases with behavior and adolescent character disturbances. The patients slept better, were quieter, more cooperative, and able to work. Clerici calls particular attention to its efficacy in cases displaying impulsive rage reactions and changes in social behavior, his dosage being 0.1 to 0.2 milligram by mouth or hypodermically, three times a day. These results however remain only as long as bulbocapnine is given; when the medication is interrupted, the old picture returns quite abruptly.

SCOPOLAMINE (HYOSCINE)

At the present time scopolamine is one of the most popular forms of medication employed in cases of postencephalitic Parkinsonism. It may be given by mouth or hypodermically. Its administration in postencephalitic Parkinsonism was first recommended by Avezzù in 1921, and also in the same year by both Babinski and Souques. Avezzù prescribed the following:

Scopolamine hydrobromide.........	0.015 gram
Aqu. dest........................	150.0 cc.

One teaspoon of this solution contains 0.00025 gram scopolamine. Avezzù ordered one teaspoon twice a day and allowed rest intervals of five to six days after twenty-five days of medication.

The difference in the effect of scopolamine upon the afflicted and the nonafflicted is remarkable. In the normal person $\frac{1}{100}$ grain produces dryness of the mouth, slight confusion, incoordination of speech, slight ataxia upon walking, and disturbances in accommodation. Every motion becomes difficult and the effect culminates in several hours of sleep. In cases of postencephalitic Parkinsonism, however, similar doses produce only slight side effects, while the salivation decreases, tremor and rigidity diminish, speaking is facilitated and the previously altered chronaxia becomes normal. Subjectively, the patient finds considerable comfort in this medication.

Schaltenbrand has discussed addiction to scopolamine. Like morphine, when the drug is stopped there are withdrawal symptoms, but without the accompany of cachexia. Schaltenbrand suggests that hyoscine be administered in the same manner as arsenic, giving increasing and decreasing doses, in a solution of 1:1000, the doses being as small as possible.

Old solutions of scopolamine become ineffective, which accounts for many inadequate results, particularly if the druggist has had the same solution for a long time. This can be avoided by employing Merck's comprettes, each of which contains 0.0001 gram hyoscine.

Hohmann began to use scopolamine in 1921, reporting on the results in eighteen cases in 1924. As a rule, $\frac{1}{100}$ grain was administered four times daily. The highest dose was $\frac{1}{50}$ grain four times a day. The side effects were negligible, the results were good, and included alleviation of some psychic symptoms. Many cases returned to work after having been invalided and bedridden for a long time. The medication, however, was without any influence upon behavior disturbances.

Patry combined hypodermic and oral administration, beginning with an injection of $\frac{1}{200}$ grain in the morning. If there are no side effects, the same dose is given by mouth at noontime and again at night. After a few days the doses both by mouth and hypodermically are increased to $\frac{1}{150}$ grain. More than $\frac{1}{50}$ grain three times a day should not be given at any one time. When side effects are very disturbing, $\frac{1}{20}$ to $\frac{1}{10}$ grain pilocarpine may be given. As is true of all alkaloid therapy, medication with hyoscine must be continued throughout a lifetime.

The question arises as to whether hyoscine may be given in large doses. Zahorski observed good effects with doses of 0.01 gram; and Patry recommends large doses combined with ultraviolet ray exposure until a strong erythema appears. I personally have been reluctant to prescribe large doses of scopolamine, as in my experience Parkinsonian patients have far less tolerance to scopolamine than to atropine. Moreover, there is always the danger of marked psychomotor excitement and hallucinations, often followed by a collapse of the vascular system.

Large doses may be tried only with the so-called genoscopolamine, an amino-oxide of hyoscine discovered by Polonovski in 1925 and zealously employed in France. Its pharmacological qualities are approximately similar to scopolamine, but the former is two hundred times less poisonous. Lados, in 1927, reported sixteen cases treated with this preparation. Beginning with 1 or 2 milligrams, the dose is rapidly increased up to 3 to 4 milligrams. Usually, the maximal dose is 4 milligrams, but there is no danger in larger doses, if the case seems to call for them.

Granules are given by mouth, each containing 0.5 milligram, or a solution of 1.5:1,000 (2 drops = 1 milligram). For hypodermic purposes, 1 ampule contains 1 milligram The result will be enhanced if the total dose is given in two or three injections in the course of the day. Genoscopolamine is not habit forming.

Before having recourse to the Bulgarian treatment, I employed with quite satisfactory results, an Italian compound, eustateina, which contains scopolamine. This preparation is distributed in two bottles; the original prescription, after Franchini is:

	per cent
Bottle no. 1:	
Acid. sclerotin	4.1
Ioscina brom.	0.063
Am. di amigdal	1.38
Verato rizoma	6.0
Bottle no. 2:	
Ioscina brom.	0.126
Idrol di prun. Laur. cer. tit.	1.38
Laurocereasina q.b.a.c.	3
Alc. rad. aconit. tit. al.	0.5
Alcaloidi totali	1.8
As. sotto forma organica	0.0013 p.c.

Twenty drops from bottle no. 1 are given in sugar water in the morning, and the same dose from bottle no. 2 at noontime.

The dose is slowly increased each day until an optimal effect is reached. The addition of veratrine increases the functional capacity of the muscles, whereas aconite decreases the sensory irritability.

Satisfactory results are commonly observed shortly after the onset of the treatment, including a favorable influence upon oculogyric crises.

ATROPINE

Nonne, in 1923, was the first to recommend atropine in the treatment of postencephalitic Parkinsonism; later Szyszka administered dosages up to 4.5 milligrams daily, effecting a diminution in salivation with improvment in motility and amimia. Since then atropine has been administered by many physicians, the first hypodermic use of it being made by Reys in Strasbourg, but the results have not proven entirely satisfactory and they are certainly not better than those previously obtained with other medications.

The picture changed when, in 1929, Anna Luise Kleemann, first assistant to Dr. Roemer at his sanitarium in Hirsau, Germany, reported on the results obtained by the use of extremely large doses of atropine. These were much larger than any hitherto administered, being ten to twenty times the maximal dose suggested in the pharmacopoeia. This treatment is now known as Roemer's method, unfortunately without reference to Dr. Kleemann.*

The rationale of large doses of atropine is based upon the

* Prof. H. W. Maier, in a discussion, at a meeting of the Neurological Society in Zurich in 1938, of my paper on the Bulgarian treatment, mentioned that in 1920 or 1921 in Zurich a charlatan treated postencephalitic Parkinsonism with great success by hypodermic injections. Later it was found that this patent medicine consisted of large doses of atropine. It follows, therefore, that a quack is the real inventor of the Kleemann-Roemer treatment.

hyposensitivity of Parkinsonians to atropine. Fleischmann, in investigations now almost forgotten (1910), demonstrated that the blood serum of rabbits is 242 times more resistant to atropine than human serum and that rabbit serum has the property of removing the toxin of atropine. He found that 1 cc. of rabbit serum will within half an hour eliminate the effect of paralysis of the vagus nerve caused by 0.005 milligram atropine. Stoorm van Leeuwen found from physiological experiments that pure atropine has a much stronger effect upon the intestine than the same dose mixed with serum. One is presumably dealing with processes of adsorption. Bremer found a considerable hyposensitivity to atropine in cases of postencephalitic Parkinsonism and stated that his experiments with the intestine showed a remarkable adsorption of atropine. On the other hand, pharmacologists do not believe that Bremer's investigations are exact, and Lewenstein has found that normal man develops a tolerance to high doses of atropine. Polkovnikova and Bouračevskij could not agree with Bremer, in the light of results which they obtained by experiments with pilocarpine upon the isolated intestine of cats.

It would seem, therefore, that a remarkable hyposensitivity to atropine exists, but this hyposensitivity cannot, at the present stage of our knowledge, be explained. Hyposensitivity to atropine is also found in traumatic injuries of the basal ganglia and in CO poisoning, but not in Parkinson's disease (paralysis agitans). On the contrary, these patients are very often extremely sensitive to atropine and also to the Bulgarian treatment, and their symptoms are often beyond influence.

That this hyposensitivity is caused by the encephalitic process can be demonstrated adequately in cases of hemiparkinsonism. Signs of poisoning such as dryness of the mouth, disturbances in accommodation and high blood pressure are quickly produced on the unaffected side by larger doses of atropine, whereas these symptoms are rarely found on the affected side, and rigidity and tremor are diminished or soon disappear. In these cases Meerloo recommends the following prescription:

	gram
Fol. bellad. pulv.	0.005
Fol. Stram. pulv.	0.015 –0.035
Gland. thyroid. pulv.	0.01 –0.02
Atrop. sulf.	0.0005–0.001
Strychnin. nitr.	0.0003
Calc. glycerinophosph.	0.1
Pulv. rad. liq. q. s. ut f. pil. No. 80	

Hyposensitivity to atropine is not a uniform phenomenon, varying with the individual and depending upon factors which have not as yet been discovered. For example, some patients are less tolerant to atropine in the morning, while infrequently other patients are hypersensitive to it and show more or less marked intoxication with doses of 4 to 6 milligrams. In such cases, one may substitute bellafolin for atropine. It is interesting that bellafolin is not only readily tolerated, but that during its administration the sensitivity to atropine decreases, so that in time bellafolin, which is prohibitive in cost, can be replaced entirely by atropine.

The method of treatment with large doses of atropine introduced by Kleemann and Roemer is still in use. The method itself is very simple. However, every patient over forty years of age must be regarded as a possible candidate for glaucoma. The oculist should therefore be consulted, and special caution is necessary in cases where the family history suggests the possibility of glaucoma.

A 0.5 per cent solution of atropine sulfate is employed, one drop being equivalent to 0.5 milligram. Treatment begins with one drop three times a day, and is increased twice daily by 1 drop. Dryness of the mouth almost invariably disappears without interruption of the medication. In cases of stomach distress, dizziness, and heart disorders, the same dose should be taken for several days prior to augmented doses. The dose is increased until no further subjective and objective improvement can be obtained, upon which the dose is decreased by 0.25 milligram twice a day until the first signs of relapse in symptoms appear. Again the dose is slightly increased until the signs of relapse have disappeared, at which point the optimal dose has been reached and is established for further treatment. Kleemann prefers to give tablets, as they are easier to take. It is also possible to administer atropine by hypodermic injections, in which case one needs only two-thirds of the dose given by mouth. The level of the optimal dose is not parallel to the severity of the disease, and medication must be continued indefinitely.

The results of Kleemann's treatment with this method of twenty-five cases for five years were as follows: 65.2 per cent were fully able to work; 21.7 per cent returned to partial work; 13.1 per cent were incapable of work. All cases were treated not only with atropine, but with massage and physical exercises. She recommends that the treatment be administered in a hospital for at least the first three or four months. Roemer himself has published his experiences in several papers, and has tried to explain the necessity of large doses. He states that the usual small doses of atropine act peripherally, while large doses influence the centers of the midbrain and diencephalon. With his opinion, that the most severe cases require the highest doses or that tolerance to atropine is determined by proximity to the onset of acute encephalitis, I find I cannot agree.

After observing that the results of atropine treatment in paralysis agitans were less effective than in postencephalitic Parkinsonism, Roemer recommended a therapeutic trial of atropine as a means of differential diagnosis. Today, we can add that not only the poor results, but also the incompatibility of atropine in these cases is of importance in differential diagnosis (von Witzleben, 1938).

According to Roemer, the effect of atropine is less toxic when the dose is increased slowly. His practice therefore is to give the same dose for several days before increasing it. It should be remembered, however, that it is impossible to have atropine-free days in the schedule, because of the profound signs of deprivation. The optimal doses given by Roemer in ninety-eight cases are shown in Table 4.

The prognosis in cases which show none or little improvement within four to six weeks is obviously unfavorable.

To be effective, atropine should be administered at regular intervals in order to guarantee a uniform content of it in the blood stream. The interval between the last night dose and the first morning dose should therefore not be too great. This condition can be met by giving the evening dose at 10 or 11 p.m. When the dose is increased, it should be done with the night dose.

TABLE 4

NUMBER OF CASES	OPTIMAL DOSE	FREQUENCY OF DOSAGE
	milligrams	
30	5	Thrice daily
40	10	Thrice daily
14	15	Thrice daily
11	20	Thrice daily
3	Over 20	Thrice daily

TABLE 5

EFFECTS	NUMBER OF TIMES
None	23
Dryness	59
Nausea and vomiting	46
Dizziness	24
Bladder disturbances	12
Heart trouble	16
Mental disorders	15

Table 5 gives Roemer's observations on the side effects of atropine treatment.

Hall records a case with extremely high temperature from which the patient died, showing symptoms similar to those in heat stroke. Spells of tachypnea and choreatic-athetotic movements are signs of overdosage. Constipation often occurs and is due to delayed peristalsis.

It should be pointed out that there are some mental disturbances which are due not to the encephalitis but to the atropine. Fatigue, lack of impulse, sleepiness, psychomotor restlessness, states of depression and paranoid delusions are the phenomena one finds. Patients have a tendency to become anxious and suspicious, and delusions and hallucinations may occur. It is important that these symptoms be recognized as being due to the atropine, for decrease in dosage is urgently indicated. It may be mentioned at this point that mental disturbances due to encephalitis almost invariably fail to react favorably to atropine. Lewenstein reports the

TABLE 6

	BEFORE TREATMENT	AFTER TREATMENT
	per cent	*per cent*
Requiring nursing	24 (49)	8 (0)
Absolutely unable to work	40 (30)	8 (13)
Partially able to work	36 (21)	72 (21)
Fully able to work		12 (65)

occurrence of mental disturbances caused by atropine, and states that the drug is contraindicated in arteriosclerosis, kidney diseases and hypertension. Ehrenberg, in contrast to Roemer, believes that thyrotoxic tachycardia is a contraindication.

Table 6 gives Lewenstein's results of atropine treatment of twenty-five patients, compared with the corresponding percentages of Roemer's results (given in parentheses).

Lewenstein is convinced that hospitalization for several months is desirable and that the best results from atropine treatment are obtained when it is combined with physical exercises. He states that the first signs of improvement appear two to three weeks after treatment is begun, and that the "automatic disturbances" (Economo), such as compulsive yawning, screaming spells, and mimic tics, tics of the tongue (Oesterreicher), spasm of the eye lids, salivation and rigidity, are the first to diminish. He finds it difficult, however, to influence the tremor.

My own experience with this treatment forces me to disagree with Lewenstein's observations. In all my cases which were treated with atropine as well as in those in which the Bulgarian treatment was used, rigidity, salivation and tremor were influenced first, while the effect on the so-called automatic disturbances appeared later. In many cases the tremor cannot be abolished to any degree, for though it improves and sometimes disappears, the tremor readiness remains and the shaking returns, as for example, following psychic irritations. Stern, Busse, and others have had the same experience. The oculogyric crises can be markedly improved, though one must admit that they are also accessible to suggestion. Nevertheless, atropine seems to have an objective influence upon this phenomenon. It has been found that hyperkinesia, psychomotor symptoms, and behavior disorders cannot be improved, even by the use of extremely large doses of the drug.

Marinesco and Façon have had good results without untoward effects in cases of torsion spasm and oculogyric crises. Contrary to other authors, they state that it is often possible to reduce the optimal dosage without compromising the degree of improvement. In some cases as long as three months and more are required for stabilization on optimal dosage, which is one reason why Roemer prefers that the patients be treated in a hospital, a preference which this author shares with him. It must be acknowledged, however, that outpatients can also be treated with some success (Hagström, Neal, Stemplinger).

There is little doubt that the atropine treatment, as introduced by Kleemann and Roemer, represents great progress in the treatment of postencephalitic Parkinsonism. On the other hand, the literature is not without statements with regard to some dangers of the treatment. Thus, for example, none of Grewel's patients recovered sufficiently to be able to work fully, and some, especially the elderly ones, developed paranoid and hallucinatory psychoses. Sahlgren has observed disturbances of the stomach and intestine, such as diarrhea or constipation, nausea, vomiting, and severe emaciation; disturbances of speech and deglutition, as well as paresis of the facial and hypoglossus nerves have also been observed, the latter sometimes occurring in cases treated with doses of atropine as small as 8 to 9 milligrams.

The question arises as to whether or not the use of large doses of such a powerful drug continued over a period of years is harmless to the organism. Siegmund reports a case in which, following medication with atropine for three years, using a dose of 12.5 milligrams daily, the patient suddenly died, showing the clinical picture of ileus. Autopsy showed a megacolon (from the ascending colon to the anus) and an enlarged stomach. In 1935, Siegmund described three more cases with the same picture.

As a result of this, Fehsenmeier conceived the idea of making clinical fluoroscopic examinations of all patients treated with atropine. In all cases she found typical phenomena, such as constipation, meteorism, lack of free HCl, and diminution in total acidity. Frequently the dilatation of the stomach and intestine were enormous, sometimes being five times the normal size.

Precise interpretation of these findings, however, is quite difficult. One cannot attribute the phenomena to the action of the drug, since the investigations of Hess and Faltischek have shown that similar alterations in the intestine and stomach are also present in cases of untreated postencephalitic Parkinsonism. It is Buscaino's belief that all cases of postencephalitic Parkinsonism show chronic changes of the intestine and that consequently atropine depresses motility and secretion more in a Parkinsonian than in a healthy person. We are, therefore, justified in assuming that the stomach and intestines of patients with postencephalitic Parkinsonism are already altered by the disease itself and may be further injured by atropine.

Brednow's X-ray examinations before and four weeks following atropine treatment showed marked changes. After the treatment the stomach was large and atonic, the plicae mucosae very clear and prominent, the motor tone weak, the movements rare and retarded, and the pylorus spastically contracted.

The foregoing shows that there is some danger in the atropine treatment and that in some cases it may be fatal. Every case should therefore be examined very carefully before the treatment is begun and control fluoroscopic examinations should be made from time to time, as long as atropine treatment is continued.

Several attempts have been made to substitute for atropine similar but less toxic medications or mixtures. Three of these preparations—apoatropine, syntropan, and rabellon—deserve description.

Apoatropine was discovered by Ladenburg in 1880. It is uncertain whether it exists in the roots of Atropa belladonna or whether it appears during the chemical and pharmacological extraction. The transformation from atropine to apoatropine occurs by splitting off a molecule of water. Apoatropine has no asymmetric C atom and is therefore optically inactive. If heated, it is transformed to belladonnine. Unlike atropine, apoatropine does not affect the ends of the vagus nerve, but has a direct influence upon smooth musculature. Its effect upon the isolated intestine is five times stronger than that of atropine.

In experiments with animals, apoatropine was found to be extremely toxic; perorally it is three times more toxic than when given hypodermically, probably because it is more quickly destroyed in the tissues than in the intestine. It affects the brain and spinal cord and, in toxic doses, produces clonic-tonic spasms, epileptic seizures, and tetanic convulsions.

Duensing was the first to use apoatropine in treating patients. He found it to be much less poisonous than when used on animals, 20 to 30 milligrams being tolerated quite well. There are almost no untoward effects and they appear only when doses of 40 milligrams or more are given. In contradistinction to atropine, there is no hyposensitivity to apoatropine. The treatment is started with 1 milligram three times a day, and is increased by three times 1 milligram daily. After the tenth day it is increased by 0.5 milligram three times a day. Pills, inexplicably, are not as well tolerated as is the fluid preparation.

Duensing treated forty-four cases, with fairly inconclusive results, particularly since in some cases it became necessary to combine it with atropine.

Syntropan is the tropic acid ester of 2.2-dimethyl-3 diethylaminoproponal, and has been used chiefly as an antispasmodic. The action upon the pupils, salivation, and so forth is from a hundred to a thousand times less than that of atropine. Chiabov administered 300 milligrams of this drug daily and Ratschov 800 milligrams. Schlezinger and Alpers treated sixteen cases over a period varying from ten days to eight months and noted that the symptoms were not relieved until 1,200 milligrams daily were given. There was no improvement in five cases, while in eleven cases a varying degree of improvement was observed. The best results were obtained with doses of about 2,400 milligrams daily. It does not seem therefore that syntropan is in any way superior to other preparations and it cannot—in company with apoatropine—be recommended in the treatment of postencephalitic Parkinsonism.

Much more favorable are the results obtained with rabellon, a mixture of hyoscyamine, scopolamine, and atropine. Each tablet contains a combined amount equivalent to 0.5 milligram of total alkaloids, expressed in hyoscyamine hydrobromides. One begins with $\frac{1}{4}$ tablet, increasing gradually until the optimum individual effect is achieved. In some instances, 5 tablets three times a day or 4 tablets four times a day become necessary.

The results obtained by Vollmer, Gayle, and others are quite good; in my own experience a number of cases have been satisfactorily influenced by this drug. Rabellon and eustateina constitute the most effective artificial mixtures of alkaloids, but they do not excel the Bulgarian treatment.

Confusion and misidentification have arisen because some authors, using rabellon, speak of the Bulgarian treatment and believe that the effective substances of the roots of belladonna exist in the same proportion in rabellon. This is erroneous, because we are as yet not entirely familiar with the nature of the effective substances or with their proportions as they exist in the belladonna roots. This will be treated in greater detail in our discussion of the Bulgarian treatment. At this point I should like to emphasize that 1) rabellon is only an *artificial mixture* of three alkaloids in wholly arbitrary proportions; and, 2) rabellon is *absolutely alien to the Bulgarian treatment* and should therefore not be referred to in this manner.

A plan of treatment worked out by Lampl may be mentioned in passing, although it embraces not only atropine, but a combination of several methods of treatment.

During the treatment, the following powder is given twice a day:

	gram
Pulv. rhizom. scop. carn.	0.3
Calc. lact.	
Sacch. lact. āā	0.2

Three to six days later, fever is induced by intramuscular injections of milk, pyrifer, and so on. After six to nine fever periods, 10 cc. calcium are given every two to three days, to a total of five to ten injections. At the same time 50 to 60 drops of bellafolin are administered daily for two to three months.

Both Lampl and Wiechowski have noted in pharmacological examinations that the so-called chemically pure substances, such as atropine or scopolamine, are not as efficacious as the total extracts from the drugs. These extracts obviously require standardization, and Lampl recommends a preparation consisting of the following drugs: Scopolia atropoides, Hyoscyamus niger, Datura stramonium, Atropa belladonna, and Nicotiana rustica. From these extracts two kinds of tablets are manufactured and called Encephanyl and Striasolan. Lampl later modified his routine and started with fever therapy, at the same time giving 3 to 5 tablets Encephanyl, after food, and 4, 7, or 9 tablets of Striasolan. In addition he recommends arsenic, diathermy, strychnine, and insulin, all administered at the same time. There is little doubt that such polypharmacy has little or no value.

HARMINE (BANISTERINE)

This is a very interesting preparation, employed for the first time in postencephalitic Parkinsonism by Beringer (1926). At the same time, the pharmacologist Lewin was experimenting with a Malpighiaceae, called Banisteria caapi Spruce, used in Peru and Ecuador as a narcotic. The Indians refer to it as Aya Huasca, meaning "the dead man's wine." They drink a decoction of it which produces a profound intoxication associated with psychomotor hyperactivity. From this plant Lewin extracted an alkaloid which he called banisterine and some time later it became evident that Lewin had been dealing with a preparation which was already well known—harmine. By 1923 French authors (Clinquart, Perrot, and others) had already found that harmine and the alkaloids derived from Banisteria caapi were identical. Harmine is extracted from Peganum harmala, a plant described by Fritzsche in 1848; somewhat later Flury investigated its effects upon the central nervous system; Tappeiner (1895) and Gunn (1910) were also interested in its action. The same alkaloid is known by the name of yageine (Villalba, 1925), its chemical constitution according to Merck being:

$$C_{13}H_{12}ON_2$$

whereas Bogota's formula is:

$$C_{13}H_8N_3O$$

The use of harmine in postencephalitic Parkinsonism is due purely to accident. When Beringer was making his famous studies on mezcaline and other narcotics, Merck sent him some banisterine so that he might investigate its effect upon the mind. One of the physicians tried it on himself by injecting 0.2 gram. He soon collapsed, displaying an entirely uncontrollable tremor of the extremities. When he gave himself a smaller dose, he found that all active movements became unusually facilitated, which led to the idea of employing the preparation in cases of postencephalitic Parkinsonism.

The manner in which the alkaloid operates, and specifically whether it affects the cortex or the basal ganglia remained unknown for a long time. Beer, in experiments with animals, found that it operates in both manners, depending upon the dose employed. Following removal of the cortex, the drug does not alter the reflexes or muscle tone; upon increasing the dose, no convulsions appear, as occurs when the cortex is not removed. Beer concluded that the use of harmine in postencephalitic Parkinsonism produces an increase in the subcortical motor and psychic impulses.

Halpern's interesting experiments have finally clarified the manner in which harmine operates. He first found that scopolamine and harmine have antagonistic effects, for scopolamine diminishes the uninhibited extrapyramidal motor movements, whereas harmine excites the cortex. Harmine, therefore, improves only arbitrary movements, and the results of its use in postencephalitic Parkinsonism depend upon which condition predominates—tremor and rigidity, or akinesia and amimia. Since, in general, both groups are usually present, and scopolamine affects the former, harmine the latter, the apparent improvement in rigidity by harmine is really secondary, as it is the improved akinesia which overcomes the rigidity.

Halpern's findings explain the contradictions which many workers have noted in the results of treatment with harmine, and they also account for the better results obtained when harmine and scopolamine are combined. Halpern administered harmine to himself and noted that he became very restless, was unable to sit still, and found it necessary to walk to and fro. Movements could readily be performed; he finally became quarrelsome and attacked people on the street.

Beringer found that favorable results followed the injection of 0.02 to 0.04 gram harmine. Suppositories of 0.02 to 0.06 gram may be given, but they are sometimes without effect. When taken by mouth the drug must be in creatine-coated capsules of 0.02 to 0.04 gram each. In the first fifteen cases described by Beringer, the hypokinesia was very much improved but there was no effect upon the tremor.

Hill and Worster-Drought treated thirty-eight cases, nineteen of them perorally, and nineteen hypodermically. Sixteen of these were severe, thirteen mild, and nine light.

The following routine was employed:

Perorally:
- 0.01 gram twice a day for 7 days
- 0.02 gram twice a day for 5 days
- 0.03 gram twice a day for 3 days

Hypodermically:
- 0.02 gram every morning for 7 days
- 0.02 gram twice a day for 7 days
- 0.04 gram twice a day for 1 day

In addition to complete absence of improvement, serious side effects were observed. On the other hand, Rosenberger, Pinéas, and Schuster report much better results. Jacobi, who treated thirty cases, in some instances observed an initial increase in the tremor, which was later followed by improvement. Further improvement followed the use of larger doses. Marinesco and others report improvement in speech and rigidity but have not seen any influence upon the tremor. An increased irritability of the vestibular apparatus and a sensitization of the carotid sinus reflexes, shown by bradycardia and decreasing blood pressure, often follow the use of harmine.

Eichler was able to demonstrate objective improvement by means of the ergograph. Nevertheless, the results obtained with harmine are not very great and there are no further reports to be found in the literature. As can be seen from Halpern's investigations, the results are entirely too variable. I myself used harmine in several cases (1927), but discontinued its use because of negligible results.

STRAMONIUM

Datura stramoniium (devil's apple, *herbe des magiciens*, *Teufelskraut*) is a plant of the Solanaceae family therapeutically employed in Europe since 1762. It was first mentioned in this country by Samuel Cooper of the University of Pennsylvania in 1779. He was familiar with its poisonous qualities and employed it in the treatment of mania and epilepsy. The leaves contain several alkaloids (total 0.33 per cent). Stramonium is probably an isomer of atropine but is differentiated by another kind of crystallization and is optically levorotatory. According to Reuter, it is only a mixture of atropine, scopolamine, and hyoscyamine (similar to rabellon).

Toxic overdoses produce unusually severe mental disturbances, especially in the form of delusions and hallucinations (*visions phantastiques*, hence devil's apple). The mydriasis is less intense than that following the use of atropine, but persists for a longer time.

The treatment of postencephalitic Parkinsonism with stramonium was introduced in Paris by Juster in 1925, and several years later, in Berlin by Sternberg. Juster administered pills, each containing 0.02 gram of the drug, increasing the dosage slowly up to 10 pills a day. Excellent results were achieved, with marked improvement in rigidity and hypokinesia. In some cases Juster combined the drug with hyoscine. In 1929, Juster again reported good results. Side effects were mild and could be avoided by decreasing the optimal doses, which were 0.5 to 1.0 gram, down to 0.2 to 0.7 gram.

Sternberg, using the new preparation, reported excellent results in twenty-eight very severe cases. The single dose was always 0.1 gram, and the optimal dose was smaller than those given by Juster or Laignel-Lavastine.

The effect is not uniform and does not depend upon the severity of the clinical picture; on the contrary, there are cases in which smaller doses seem to be more effective than larger ones. In general, there is no difference in the effect of pills or suppositories, but a few singular variations have been noted. For example, some patients developed delusions when given pills; when the medication was stopped, the delusions disappeared, and did not recur when treatment was resumed with suppositories. Women reputedly show greater sensitivity to stramonium than men, and during menstruation the side effects may become extremely disagreeable.

Ordinarily, the effects of stramonium medication appear very early but in some cases—paradoxically, in mild cases—improvement is not noted until several weeks or months have passed. On the whole, however, the optimum effect is reached within three to four weeks of medication. If, after several months, good results do not appear, an increase in dosage or a change in method is mandatory; as for example, medication by suppositories instead of by pills. The effect of stramonium on paralysis agitans is never as good as on postencephalitic Parkinsonism.

Motility improves both subjectively and objectively. The movements are quicker and stronger, and the excursions larger. Walking becomes quicker, and the steps larger; the speech improves, and patients are able to speak more fluently.

Sternberg states that in his cases the tremor was much more improved than the rigidity, an experience contrary to that of other authors. The oculogyric crises became much less frequent. The restlessness was very much improved, these patients, as is well known, being unable to sit for any length of time without getting up every few minutes to walk about.

Hoedemaker and Burns have also had encouraging results

with stramonium; they state that the tremor was very much diminished. They administered a 10 per cent tincture, starting with 20 minims three times a day, increasing slowly to 60 minims or more. There is no correlation between the therapeutic effect, the severity of the disease, or its duration; generally, severe cases were much more resistant to the therapy.

There are wide differences in the dosage employed by various doctors. Worster-Drought and Hill administered a tincture (B.Ph.) which is twenty times weaker than the extract of stramonium U.S.P. They started with 20 to 30 minims and increased the dose quickly to 90 to 120 minims, or eight times the maximal dose. Large doses of the leaves often being well tolerated, they also administered dry extracts, since these have the advantage of a higher alkaloid content in less bulk. The extract (alcoholic percolate, U.S.P.) contains 1 per cent of total alkaloids, whereas the leaves contain only 0.1 to 0.7 per cent, the average content being 0.25 per cent.

A standardized tincture (U.S.P.) was tried by Jacobson and Epplen, who started with 20 minims three times a day, the average optimal dose being about 60 minims four times a day. The authors were quite content with the results, except for its effect on the tremor. But when, in addition, they injected $\frac{1}{50}$ grain hyoscine, one to two times a day, the tremor was satisfactorily influenced. Shapiro reports on sixteen cases, eleven of whom were markedly improved with respect to rigidity, salivation, posture, speech, and mental disorders. Hurst administered a combination of stramonium and pilocarpine, stating that he thus obtained much more impressive results than with stramonium alone. Hurst's initial dose was 10 drachms of tincture stramonium, three times a day, and each dose was increased every other day by 1 drachm. The dosage of pilocarpine nitrate was started with $\frac{1}{10}$ grain and increased slowly. The optimal dose was generally 60 drachms stramonium and $\frac{2}{5}$ grain pilocarpine.

Contrary to most English and American authors, (Burns,

Harris, Steen) Cottrell finds the U.S.P. tincture entirely uncertain, and prefers to administer pills, each containing $2\frac{1}{2}$ grains. Increasing doses are given, up to 3 pills three times daily.

My own experiences with stramonium cannot be considered extensive. Employing only pills and suppositories, the results obtained have been identical to those mentioned by Sternberg and others. To my surprise, improvement in some mental disorders was to be noted, as well as the appearance of a euphoria coupled with increased psychic activity. Investigations with the ergograph confirmed Carmichael and Green's comparison of the effects of hyoscine and stramonium. While improvement followed medication with stramonium, in quite a large number of cases further improvement followed when stramonium was combined with hyoscine.

THE BULGARIAN TREATMENT ACCORDING TO RAEFF, PANEGROSSI AND VON WITZLEBEN

Of all the methods of alkaloid therapy previously mentioned, large doses of atropine, administered according to Kleemann and Roemer's method seem to be the most efficacious for the treatment of postencephalitic Parkinsonism. The main disadvantage of this method, however, is that a powerful poison must be administered throughout the life of the patient, in doses ten times or more the previous maximum dose. At first there were very serious and sometimes fatal side effects, which remained unavoidable until an improved medication became available. Such a superior medication is the so-called Bulgarian treatment discovered in Bulgaria by a lay herbalist by the name of Raeff.

About fifteen years ago rumors spread all over Europe about the marvelous and surprising results which Raeff achieved in the treatment of postencephalitic Parkinsonism by the use of a secret medication. Later, it became known that this magic remedy consisted of a vinous decoction of Atropa belladonna. Since then, this treatment has been called the Bulgarian treatment, no difference in nomenclature being made, whether the decoction is obtained from Bulgarian roots or from those of any other country. Bulgarian treatment therefore refers only to the use of a total extract from the roots of Atropa belladonna. All artificial preparations or mixtures, such as rabellon, have nothing to do with the Bulgarian treatment, and it is difficult to understand why this misleading designation should continue in the literature to be applied to the use of rabellon.

Raeff's original method, with which I began my own experiments, comprised four ingredients, designated by Raeff himself as:

(1) Racine no. 1
(2) Poudre no. 2
(3) Pillules no. 3
(4) Racine no. 4

Pharmacologically these four ingredients were found to consist of:

(1) roots of belladonna
(2) charcoal
(3) bread paste, mixed with nutmeg and shavings
(4) roots of calmus

Raeff's original prescription reads as follows: Ivan Raeff—village of Schipka—Bulgaria. 30 grains of (1) together with one powder (2) are boiled (air-tight) in 600 cc. of natural white wine for ten minutes. After filtration, the fluid is drawn off and carefully corked in a bottle. This fluid is then administered as follows: Up to five years of age, ½ tablespoon is required; up to ten years, 1 tablespoon; to twenty years, 2 tablespoons; and later 3 tablespoons (daily). The total daily dose is taken at one time, and not apportioned in fractions; the medication is given during the first hours of sleep, so that it becomes necessary to awaken the patient. After three to four days, a "crisis" appears, lasting for a few hours. If the crisis is prolonged the dose must then be reduced. Each morning before breakfast a pill (3) must be taken with milk or hot tea. Every two hours (six to seven times a day) the patient should chew a piece of (4). Diet: meat is forbidden, as are pepper and sour foods, beans, peas, and any variety of alcoholic beverage.

This treatment might have continued to remain obscure and mysterious had it not been for the Queen of Italy, who instigated the scientific investigation of Raeff's preparations and their administration.

In my opinion, (1) is probably the main effective substance; (2) may have some effect on the intestine, though nothing definite has been established up to now; (3) is definitely obsolete; and (4) is useful in producing saliva and diminishing dry throat. In my own experience, the content of alkaloids decreases if Raeff's charcoal is added to the decoction; this is especially true with carbo medicinalis Merck. For example, a vinous decoction of 16.3 milligrams per cent alkaloids decreases to 15.6 milligrams per cent upon the addition of Raeff's powder. Upon the addition of Merck's charcoal, alkaloid can no longer be found. The therapeutic effect continues to be as excellent without charcoal as with it.

The main alkaloids so far identified in the roots of Atropa belladonna are hyoscyamine (80 to 90 per cent), scopolamine, atropine, and belladonine. Duboisine, mentioned by Panegrossi and others, is merely a mixture of hyoscinamine and scopolamine. Scopolamine is sometimes missing or found only in very small quantities, i.e., 0.1 milligram. The so-called by-alkaloids are not yet well known.

There is little doubt that Raeff's decoction is a powerful poison and should not be administered in the uncertain and inexact manner that he outlined. It is no wonder that severe "crises" (obviously nothing more than toxic poisoning) and fatal untoward effects occurred. Whether an alcoholic extract, as employed by Raeff, is of any further advantage, is unknown. Perhaps the alcohol is a preservative, but it has no influence as a therapeutic agent.

The question soon arose as to whether only the roots of Bulgarian belladonna alone are effective or whether those of other countries could also be employed. There is some difference between the Italian and Bulgarian root, the former being without odor, cylindricfusiform, not very fleshy, brown-yellow with brown-reddish tranverse processes and lengthy whitish spots. The Bulgarian root has the odor of mint, is of a dirty-white color, wrinkled, and with yellow tranverse processes (Ferrannini).

Most authors believe that there is no great difference between the Italian roots and those of other countries, as far as the therapeutic effect is concerned. Nannizzi has shown that special factors are indispensable for the production of a powerful preparation. The best plants grow in moist forests of the subalpine zone, at an altitude of 600 to 1,800 meters (2,400 to 5,400 feet). If one cultivates Italian belladonna in Bulgaria under the same conditions as the Bulgarian plants, the Italian plant becomes entirely similar to the Bulgarian. The content of alkaloids varies and is dependent upon altitude, moisture, sunshine, time of harvest, kind of soil, and other factors. The alkaloid content of very young and very old plants is not as great as that of plants two to three years old, at which age the alkaloid content seems to be greatest. The time of harvest is important, though there seems to be no agreement as to the exact time. The Italian pharmacopeia recommends harvest while the plant is in flower, while others believe that the content of the alkaloids is extremely low at that time. Cultivated plants, as on the plain of Pavia, are sometimes better than wild ones.

Panegrossi found the total content of alkaloids in the Bulgarian roots to be about 0.86 per cent, in the root stock 0.5 per cent. Ceni states that the Bulgarian root is richer in the active principle than the Italian.

In my own experience the roots purchased from Raeff contained 0.87 per cent total alkaloids, or twice that of roots received from other Bulgarian firms. The French and German roots also contain only about 0.5 per cent. Fabing has made a comparison of the American and Italian roots by preparing a decoction using an American white wine with an alcohol content of 13.5 per cent. He found the Bulgarian decoction to contain 0.0208 per cent, while the American contained 0.0295 per cent of alkaloids. Paradoxically, the alkaloids content does not parallel the therapeutic effect. For example, the Indian root contains 1.65 per cent and yet it does not have a therapeutic effect superior to the Bulgarian root. I have noted that extracts of Bulgarian and German roots with exactly the same alkaloids content had a different effect, the Bulgarian root being decidedly more powerful. There is as yet no final decision as to which root is superior, and further and more extensive investigation is needed along this line. Unfortunately, in some European countries, national and commercial interests are decisive in the choice of medication.

To avoid the disadvantages inherent in Raeff's decoction, the preparation of tablets possessing a uniform alkaloid content was recommended, though in my opinion tablets per se are inferior to fluid extracts. The dilution and absorption of tablets in the intestine is more dependent upon individual and local circumstances than, for example, that of a fluid extract which can be administered in the form of drops.

Though some authors are convinced that the so-called chemically "pure" alkaloids would be therapeutically satisfactory if administered in the same proportions in which they exist in the belladonna roots (rabellon), as yet, not all the alkaloids existing in the roots nor the proportions in which they appear are known. Practical experience soon demonstrated that such mixtures were inferior to the genuine total extracts (Lampl, Neal and Dillenberg, Kauders and Oesterreicher, von Witzleben).

Initial progress in the administration of the decoction was made by Panegrossi, who succeeded in making a cold-water extraction from the roots, thus avoiding the expensive alcohol.

This preparation, used in the Encephalitis Clinic in Rome, has a titer of 0.2 per cent of total alkaloids. It would seem that the alcohol contributes no advantages and does not facilitate the resorption, as believed by Kauders and Oesterreicher.

Panegrossi starts his treatment with 1 to 2 cc., increasing by similar amounts until the optimal dose is reached. Unlike Raeff, he divides the total daily dose, distributing it over a period of twenty-four hours. The largest dose is given at night, so that if side effects such as dry throat appear, they should not interfere with the patient's sleep. In my opinion, the main purpose of the large dose at night is to militate against a too rapid reduction of the alkaloids content in the blood during the night interval.

If the patient does not tolerate the preparation, it may be given as an enema for the first few days.

After I had had the opportunity to study Panegrossi's method in Rome, I began to search for a standardized preparation which could be administered in the form of drops. At first, I used another Italian preparation named panatropa, which is dispensed in pills of egglike form, each containing 0.00125 gram alkaloids. The results were less gratifying than with the Panegrossi preparation, the pills being not as well tolerated as fluids, and an exact dosage with pills being impossible.

In collaboration with a chemical firm in Switzerland I finally succeeded in producing a standardized total extraction of belladonna roots. After many experiments we decided to use only Bulgarian roots because of substantially better results. This preparation we called "Bulgakur" (in Germany, "Homburg 680"). One drop contains 0.075 milligram of total alkaloids, 40 drops equalling 1 cc. or 3 milligrams of total alkaloids. The bottle is calibrated, assuring exact dosage.

There is no routine schedule for the administration of Bulgakur or any other preparation of belladonna roots, and each case must be treated individually to determine the optimal dose. The routine described by Petrò is very dangerous and should never be used. He divides his patients into two groups: (1) those with rigidity, whom he treats with a maximal dose of 60 cc. daily, and (2) those with tremor, whom he treats with a maximal dose of 90 cc. daily.

In general, the Bulgakur treatment is started with one drop of the medication, which is given in the evening. The increase of dosage is shown in Table 7. In many cases one may increase the doses more rapidly. The average dose is 15 to 25 drops three times a day. In a few cases it is necessary to give an additional dose during the night, as the night interval is too long for some patients. Very sensitive patients should be given the total dose in four fractions instead of three.

TABLE 7

Bulgakur dosage

DAY	MORNING	NOON	EVENING
	number of drops	*number of drops*	*number of drops*
1st	—	—	1
2nd	—	1	1
3d	1	1	1
4th	1	1	2
5th	1	2	2
6th	2	2	2

Scheiffarth gives the same dose every four hours and a larger dose at bedtime, by which means he thinks a more uniform effect is achieved. The dose at bedtime is four times as high as the single diurnal dose to be given the following day. For example, when the night dose is 4 drops, the dose on the following day is 1 drop given four times. In no case did he use more than 40 drops, the equivalent of 3 milligrams total alkaloids.

If patients have been treated with atropine prior to the inception of the Bulgarian treatment, the change must be effected gradually and cautiously. A sudden transition from one drug to the other cannot be recommended. If, for example, the patient has had 4 milligrams atropine four times daily, the last dose at night is the first to be replaced by 10 drops

Bulgakur; after one or two days, the noon dose and the following morning dose are changed in the same manner, so that the patient receives 10 drops three times daily. From then on the dose is increased in the usual manner.

As to the stability of the preparation, Panegrossi has demonstrated that his decoction retains a uniform alkaloids content for a long time; Gandellini has found that after thirty to thirty-five days the total alkaloids content decreased slightly, but that the therapeutic effect was unchanged. There seems to be no doubt that the alkaloids content is not constant, being variable even in the root and dependent upon the humidity. The Italian root, seven times as moist as the Bulgarian root, dries more rapidly, with a resultant loss in alkaloids, whereas in the Bulgarian roots the alkaloids are almost invariable and constant. Though Bulgakur is prepared in a special manner, to avoid changing the effective levorotatory hyoscyamine into optically inactive substances, experiments nevertheless show that there is a slight diminution in alkaloids content after a few months have elapsed. This change in content is so small as to make little difference in treatment. However, when Bulgakur is transferred to other climates, as for example from Europe to a hot climate, the total alkaloids seem to diminish after a few weeks and the therapeutic effect is not as good.

Side effects in the Bulgarian treatment are similar to those of atropine, but they are, especially when Bulgakur is used, much milder and appear later, because the doses of alkaloids needed for a sustained therapeutic effect are smaller. There is some dryness of the throat (xerostomia), accompanied by thirst and difficulty in deglutition. Blurring of vision due to disturbances of accommodation occurs, and sometimes dizziness and a slightly elevated temperature. Nausea, vomiting, diarrhea or constipation, and disturbances of the bladder are not often seen.

These side effects, when they occur, can be readily controlled. Eserine is effective for dryness of the throat and for bladder trouble (combined with applications of heat to the bladder area). Pilocarpine diminishes the blurring of vision. When the patient's optimal dose has been established and administered for at least three to four weeks, the disturbed accommodation may be corrected by glasses. Ice pills are useful in case of vomiting, or Bulgakur may be given rectally for some time. In all cases in which the side effects appear to be harmless, it is better to avoid any interruption of the treatment, but the dose should be decreased by one-fifth or one-fourth.

Panegrossi has not had any fatalities as a consequence of the treatment, nor have I. Giugni, however, states that the treatment renders the patient more susceptible to infectious diseases.

Certain contraindications should be recalled at this point. Cardiac diseases accompanied by insufficiency do not necessarily constitute a contraindication, provided the insufficiency can be properly treated, as, for example, with strophanthin. Caution must be exercised, however, in cases of aortic syphilis and angina pectoris. Syphilis should not be treated with arsphenamin or similar preparations because of the clinical incompatibility between arsenic and Bulgakur. Glaucoma is almost invariably a contraindication to treatment, and no such case should be treated prior to careful examination by an ophthalmologist. Furthermore, large doses of pilocarpine should be administered in such instances. There has never been a case of postencephalitic Parkinsonism complicated by glaucoma in my personal experience.

Pulmonary tuberculosis does not constitute a contraindication if the process is fibrous and nonulcerative; otherwise great caution is necessary.

Various liver disturbances are frequently associated with chronic encephalitis. Tests to evaluate liver function should be made and if it is found that the damage is minor, treatment may be attempted.

Severe prostatic hypertrophy as well as kidney insufficiency constitute contraindications. Similarly, cases showing extreme exhaustion and cachexia should also not be treated.

Occasionally, signs of acute encephalitis appear, such as rise in temperature and somnolence. These symptoms are a strict contraindication to further therapy.

Irritable and excited psychopathic personalities should not be treated or, if treated, given only small doses. Epilepsy due to the encephalitis may be treated, but the so-called genuine epilepsy is a strict contraindication.

Stomach and intestines should be roentgenologically examined prior to and periodically during the treatment in order not to overlook the development of a dangerous state of megacolon. Strangely enough, changes in the stomach and intestines due to encephalitis found prior to treatment are not further aggravated by the Bulgarian treatment.

TABLE 8

Results of Bulgarian treatment by Panegrossi

	MILD CASES	MODERATE CASES	SEVERE CASES
	per cent	*per cent*	*per cent*
Virtually cured	60	49.2	14.6
Markedly improved	26	36.1	48.1
Improved	14	14.02	37.2
Not improved	0	0.68	0.1

Hypertension and old age are not contraindications to therapy. Pregnancy may be treated with little danger. Panegrossi has never observed untoward results, although belladonna is secreted in the mother's milk and can be found in the child's urine.

With regard to the results of Bulgarian treatment, Panegrossi's experience stands in first place, since up to now he has treated the greatest number of cases, a total of 1,968 cases from 1934 to 1939 (Table 8). He classifies his cases as mild, moderate, severe and extremely severe. In mild cases there is some hypertonus, unilateral for the most part, which may or may not be combined with slight hyperkinesia, with consequent reduction in working ability. Moderate cases have similar but more intensified symptoms and are unable to work at all.

In severe and extremely severe cases there is complete akinesia and complete loss of movement; patients are bedridden and dependent upon nursing care.

Panegrossi considers a patient "Virtually recovered" if he shows slight defects but is able to resume his work. He states that his best results have been in mild cases which show slow progress and have had no previous treatment. But the contrary is also seen (which corresponds with my own experience), in that severe cases improve more than anticipated, whereas mild cases often show little or no improvement. I have been unable to verify the statement of Levi-Bianchini and others that compatibility and effect are proportionate to the duration and severity of the disease.

My own results with the Bulgarian treatment of 827 cases are given in Table 9. I have classified as mild cases those who, though having to be hospitalized, are still able to care for themselves (eating, dressing); as moderate cases have been listed those up and about, but having some difficulty in feeding themselves and generally requiring nursing care; while cases have been classified as severe when almost entirely akinetic, rigid, and requiring special care.

As can be noted from the table, the total number of practically cured and markedly improved is far above that claimed by Roemer or reached by any other therapy employed. Indeed, very severe cases who have been bedridden for a long time display very marked improvement.

This has been true in spite of the fact that only comparatively small doses need be administered, in contrast to the extremely large doses of atropine employed by the Roemer method. From the social point of view, particularly, it is significant that 71 per cent of all cases succeeded in returning to work.

All of the symptoms are not equally influenced, so that prior to treatment it is difficult to determine the degree of improvement to be anticipated. Generally speaking, the first improvement can be observed within two or three weeks of the start

TABLE 9

Total number: 827. Male: 671 (81.14%). Female: 156 (18.86%).

	PERCENT	NUMBER	ABLE TO WORK	PERCENTAGE
Mild cases: 236 (28.53% of total number)				
Practically cured	58	137	137	100
Very marked improvement	26	61	61	100
Marked improvement	12	28	28	100
Moderate improvement	3	7	3	43
Not improved	1	2	0	0
Moderate cases: 282 (34.09%)				
Practically cured	45	127	127	100
Very marked improvement	31	87	85	97.7
Marked improvement	14	39	30	76.9
Moderate improvement	6	17	2	11.7
Not improved	4	11	1	9.
Severe cases: 309 (37.36%)				
Practically cured	9	28	21	75
Very marked improvement	43	133	81	61
Marked improvement	28	87	14	16
Moderate improvement	13	40	0	0
Not improved	7	22	0	0
Percentage calculated according to the total number of cases:				
Practically cured	37	292	285	97.0
Very marked improvement	33	282	227	80.5
Marked improvement	18	154	72	46.7
Moderate improvement	7	64	5	7.8
Not improved	4	35	1	2.8

	ABLE TO WORK	
	Percent	Number
Mild cases	97.3	230
Moderate cases	86.8	245
Severe cases	37.6	116
Total		591 (71%) of total number (827)

of treatment; then the progress slows down and sometimes months are required until the optimal dose is reached.

Best influenced are the symptoms of rigidity and amimia, bradykinesia, catalepsy, walking, speech, deglutition, and handwriting. These improvements can be objectively verified, for example, by means of a kymograph. The cogwheel rigidity improves or disappears as does Soederberg's myodystonic reaction. Furthermore, there is some relationship between muscle hypertony, creatine, and the amount of creatinine in the urine. The more marked the improvement, the less creatine is found in the urine.

As far as the tremor and other hyperkinesias are concerned, the results obtained vary widely. Tremor may disappear, but in almost all cases a tremor readiness remains. Benvenuti, Gandellini, and myself among others, have observed that tremor which was not previously present may appear at the beginning of treatment. The reason for this is not known. Panegrossi believes that the tremor is produced by the rapid diminution of the rigidity, an assumption which supports the previously mentioned relationship between tremor and rigidity (Jackson). In such cases, the tremor disappears if the dose is increased.

Pain, paresthesia, and contractures of muscles are improved, whereas true deformities of the joints are not.

Oculogyric crises are favorably influenced by the treatment, as are also the compulsive symptoms often associated with these crises. Generally speaking, all varieties of tics and myoclonic movements of the extremities, face, and tongue improve, but torsion spasm and athetosis are quite resistant and sometimes cannot be influenced at all.

I have not observed satisfactory results in cases with epileptic seizures due to the encephalitic process (the so-called subcortical or extrapyramidal epilepsy).

Though Panegrossi has found improvement in the well-known sensitivity of postencephalitics to climate and inclement weather, I cannot confirm it from my own experience.

In cases with functional disturbances of the liver, Caramazza has noted the disappearance of pathologic urinary findings and a return to normal of the Weltmann reaction, following one year of treatment.

Such disturbances in water balance as oliguria and polyuria may become ameliorated with therapy.

In contradistinction to the satisfactory results mentioned, such symptoms related to the acute stage of the disease as facial paresis, nystagmus, and so on remain uninfluenced.

There is considerable discussion concerning the influence of the Bulgarian treatment upon psychic disturbances and the development of true psychoses. There is no doubt that the general affect is heightened, often approaching euphoria. Benvenuti has noted an improvement in depressed states, in emotional rigidity, and even in states of psychomotor excitement with optic and auditory hallucinations and paranoid trends. Those with deeply rooted character disturbances (asocial criminals) invariably have a poor prognosis and become worse, especially if such disturbances are combined with motor excitement. Meco's experience of four such cases, which improved markedly in spite of the long duration of symptoms, is therefore unique.

A very small percentage of patients, according to Panegrossi 0.8 per cent, do not tolerate the medication, and treatment must therefore be curtailed. When the intolerance occurs at a later stage of the treatment, it is almost always due to a disregard on the part of the patient of the prohibition of alcohol or tobacco. Tolerance of the treatment also varies with the time of year. In summer, the Bulgarian treatment is often poorly tolerated and the dose should be reduced correspondingly. This is of great importance, as otherwise a patient with symptoms of heat stroke may die during treatment.

Combination with other remedies should be avoided, except for benzedrine in isolated cases (Disertori).

Following discharge of the patient from the hospital, Bulgarian treatment must be continued at home in the manner outlined. Contrary to atropine medication however, it is possible in many cases to reduce the dose without impairing the results. Printed instructions, given to the patient when he is discharged from the hospital, will help to avoid relapses.

In spite of numerous experiments and investigations, the mechanism of the Bulgarian treatment is not yet understood. The main questions are: Does it act upon the neurovegetative system only or does it also act upon the extrapyramidal motor system? Does it influence the sympathetic system, the parasympathetic system or both? Does it act peripherally or centrally? Is it irritating or paralyzing?

Ceni demonstrated a paralyzant effect upon both the sympathetic and parasympathetic systems, but predominantly upon the latter. Though no histological changes were found in the brain and spinal cord, it does not necessarily preclude any effects upon the central nervous system. Perhaps the substantia nigra is influenced by the medication, possibly through the vessels and their nerves.

Marinesco states that the treatment acts by changing the vagus tone, which is heightened in postencephalitis. There is, moreover, a direct influence upon the muscles, as proven by the changes in chronaxia. Most authors believe in a double effect, peripheral as well as central.

The literature on the Bulgarian treatment is quite extensive, and for the most part, it reports good results obtained with Panegrossi's remedy or with other decoctions. There are two preparations in use in the United States which are worthy of mention: Bellabulgara and Bulgadonna. Bellabulgara is the name of an extract of Bulgarian belladonna root, put up by Lederle in New York. The preparation is in tablet form. Each tablet contains 0.4 milligram in total alkaloids content, and is equivalent to approximately 2 cc. of the original decoction. Neal and Maybarduk report good results with this medication.

Bulgadonna is a vinous decoction of Bulgarian belladonna roots put up by Lascoff in New York, and contains 0.16 milligram total alkaloids per cc. So far, the cases treated with this preparation have reacted very favorably.

My own results, as described above, have been obtained with Bulgakur. Since then, several others have verified the value of this preparation (Hechler, Scheiffahrth, Schmitz, Strauch). Schmitz states that he found remarkable improvement in mental disorders, such as he has never been able to obtain with any other preparation.

At this point I should like to emphasize again one aspect of the treatment, namely, that the best results are obtained only in combination with physical exercises, described in the following chapter. It is my firm belief that this combination, introduced by me several years ago, has produced noteworthy progress in the treatment of postencephalitic Parkinsonism.

It should be realized that the application of the Bulgarian treatment is not as simple as it at first seems. Good results are the product of experience in administering treatment and patience on the part of both physician and patient.

In consequence of the excellent results obtained, the Bulgarian treatment must now be considered the treatment of choice in postencephalitic Parkinsonism. There are no longer any mixtures or "pure" alkaloids which are active competitors. According to Neal and Dillenberg, "the results of Bulgarian treatment are far superior to those of rabellon . . . and to those obtained with any other form of symptomatic treatment." This statement is all the more valuable in that all the patients treated by Neal were outpatients.

OUTLINE OF TREATMENT BY PHYSICAL EXERCISES AND CALISTHENICS

Chapter 12

OUTLINE OF TREATMENT BY PHYSICAL EXERCISES AND CALISTHENICS

As repeatedly observed, motor disturbances constitute the paramount symptom in postencephalitic Parkinsonism. It is obvious, therefore, that these must be treated by special methods which will supplement the Bulgarian treatment. The contributory value of calisthenics was first recognized by Roemer who sedulously employed this method in his sanitarium. The treatment is extremely protracted and laborious, requiring great patience on the part of both patient and instructor. The service of an expert instructor is essential. Physician and instructor must be mutually reliant, particularly, because the physician is, all too often, quite unversed in the instructor's art.

Each case should be analyzed very carefully by both physician and instructor in order to avoid the disappointments which are sure to result from improperly planned therapy. These desiderata originate from my experience in many hundreds of cases and from an intimate collaboration for almost seven years with a highly specialized instructor.

Careful selection of patients is a cardinal rule. Very severe bedridden cases must be treated at first solely with massage and Bulgakur. Severe contractures should never be put in plaster bandages, a step which, contrary to treatment in spastic paresis, is extremely harmful. In all such cases the orthopedist should be consulted.

Tremor and other forms of hyperkinesia prove much more resistant to this method of treatment than cases with prevailing hypertonic-akinetic symptoms. Severe retropulsion and propulsion can be seriously obstructive, especially if there is dropped foot. Weil witnessed good results by supporting the heel with an artificial heel of approximately 5 centimeters. In cases of propulsion, the forefoot must be supported.

Because of the susceptibility of most patients to music and kindred rhythms, these may be employed to great advantage (Meyer, Treves and Treves). Moreover, these patients often develop devices to cope with symptoms which are particularly disturbing to them. Some of these tricks are very strange and their efficacy cannot be explained. Astwazaturow mentions a patient who, seated, found great difficulty in rising. The patient devised the following trick: he crossed his legs; uncrossing them immediately, he could get up with ease. Other patients to whom this trick was recommended adopted it with success. One patient who had experienced great difficulty in walking, discovered that small impediments, such as pieces of wood, which he had to step over, improved his gait. He therefore fixed to the bottom of his cane a transverse metal bar over which he stepped.

It is well known that patients with oculogyric crises and torsion spasm successfully employ many tricks. Spasms of the eyelids, for example, cease when the mouth is opened to its widest extent (similar to Gunn's syndrome).

Simple baths, beginning with a temperature of 99.1 F. and increasing to 102 F. or 103 F., when given two or three times a week for fifteen to twenty minutes, are helpful in decreasing the rigidity. The combination of massage and exercise while the patient is in the water, corresponding to the underwater treatment of poliomyelitis, is beneficial. It is certain that massage is very useful, but it must be applied correctly. Percussion massage and muscle lifting or clipping should never be used. Only a mild friction massage is permissible.

Physical exercises are performed both actively and passively. The possibility of active flexion and stretching of an extremity is first tested. If full flexion is impossible, passive help is given; or it may be advisable to first carry out the passive movement, which is then repeated actively by the patient. Short, distinct commands and a gong are aids in doing these exercises, especially if the patient has to relearn compound movements, which a healthy person does spontaneously, (writing, piano playing, buttoning and unbuttoning garments, and so on). Very often the treatment of torticollis or torsion spasm with massage and physical exercises is unsuccessful. These patients are very sensitive to irritations of any kind.

In getting postencephalitics to perform physical exercises and calisthenics one difficulty is frequently encountered; although the patients retain the faculty of concentration and the will to oblige, it is impossible for them to acquiesce due to an insurmountable inhibition. Each such situation is exceptional to the patient, similar to the "exceptional situation" (Goldstein) in cases of aphasia. On the other hand, movements are uninhibited if the patient is not forced to enact these motions with his full attention. For example, if a patient is unable to supinate and pronate the forearm on command, he is asked to toss a tennis ball and catch it as it comes down. In this manner, which we may term the "principle of detour," he successfully performs supination and pronation.

Calisthenics should therefore be started at first in the form of play, with instruction in playing. The difficulty of the play can then be gradually increased. The following equipment is useful: hoops, rope, handballs of graduated sizes, large balls (so-called medicine balls), rings, Indian clubs, and gymnastic wands. Two examples will illustrate the manner in which the equipment is used.

(1) A patient who has difficulty in walking and running must re-establish rhythm, and to this end is required to skip over, without intermediate steps, a series of balls resting at unequal intervals in a straight line. Rhythms appear as – – ⌣⌣, ⌣⌣ –, or ⌣⌣⌣, and so on.

(2) Exercises to open and close the hands are very important. The patient, seizing an Indian club at the thick end, slowly relaxes his grasp until the club is held at the neck. The neck being much thinner, the hands execute the required motions: expansion and contraction.

When the patient has mastered these exercises, he is introduced to competitive group performances, in order to spur his interest. Finally, "pure calisthenics," without equipment also based upon the principle of detour, are employed. These calisthenics are usually performed with patients prone on the floor or seated on stools, to avoid exertion, incorrect load and useless tensions. For example: to obtain flexion and stretching of the cervical vertebral column, the patient, lying on his abdomen on the floor with clasped hands at rest under his chin alternately touches his hands with forehead and chin.

Commonly, therefore, a lesson in exercises and calisthenics proceeds as follows: walking and running exercises, in straight and curved procession, are first performed. These exercises are interrupted by commands to stand still, to alter direction to squat, and so forth, which are to be obeyed as summarily as possible. After exercises with equipment and pure calisthenics are performed, the lesson concludes with a competitive game. If the weather is favorable, the lessons are given in the open air, in the shade, and, of course, with the patients clad in bathing suits.

We are deeply impressed with the results obtained by this method. It is true that hyperkinesias do not react very favorably, but rigidity and bradykinesia, as well as depressions and other mental disorders due to the chronic encephalitic process, are very much improved. Following discharge from the hospital, the majority of the patients have sufficient intelligence and insight to continue the exercises at home.

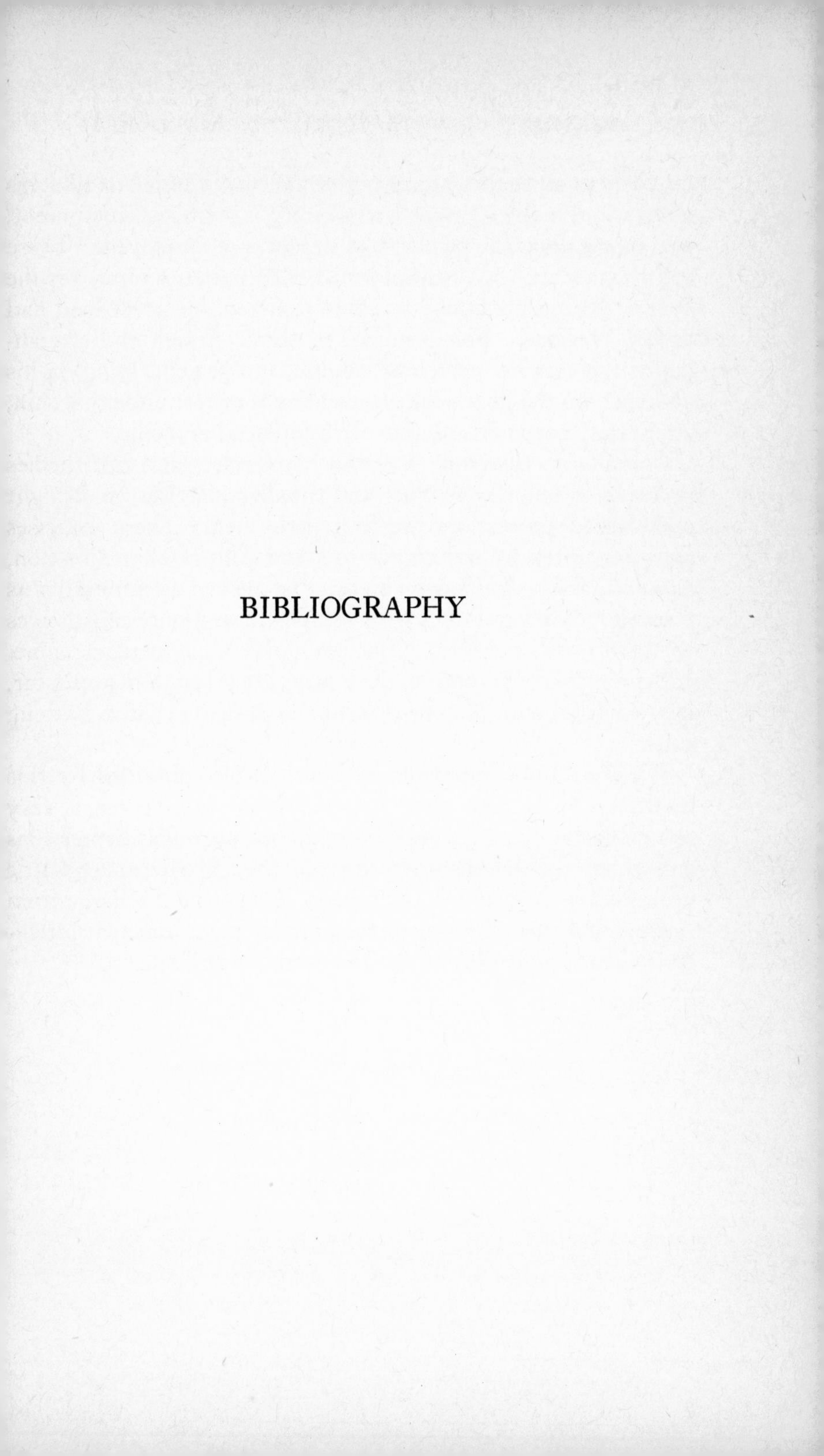

BIBLIOGRAPHY

BIBLIOGRAPHY

ABRAMSON, J. L., AND VICTOR, G. Influenza vaccine in the treatment of chronic encephalitis. J. Lab. & Clin. Med. **20:** 1043, 1935.

ADAM, S. Über günstige Erfolge von Schwefelinjektionen bei Spätencephalitis. Klin. Wchnschr. **4:** 1882, 1925.

ADAMS, F. M., AND HAYS, P. L. Treatment of the postencephalitic Parkinsonian syndrome. J. Oklahoma State M. A. **24:** 261, 1931.

ADAMS, F. M., AND HAYS, P. L. The atropine treatment of the postencephalitic Parkinsonian syndrome. Am. J. Psychiat. **91:** 151, 1934.

ADSON, A. W. Ramisection. Minnesota Med. **8:** 275, 1925.

AGOSTINI, C. La cura Bulgara del parkinsonismo postencefalitico. Policlinico (sez. prat.) **43:** 1244, 1936.

AIAZZI MANCINI, M. Contributi sperimentali all'interpretazione del meccanismo di azione della cura bulgara. Rassegna di studi psichiat. **28:** 133, 1939.

ALCOCK, N. S., AND CARMICHAEL, E. A. Investigations into treatment of Parkinsonism with Bulgarian belladonna. Quart. J. Med. **31:** 565, 1938.

ALESSANDRINI, P., AND FRATTALI, F. Le iniezioni endorachidee di solfato di magnesio nel parkinsonismo encefalitico. Bull. e Atti d. r. Acad. med. d. Roma. **52:** 242, 1926.

ALLEN, E. V., WILBUR, D. L., AND MACLEAN, A. R. Clinical experience with benzedrine sulphate. J. A. M. A. **108:** 587, 1937.

ALLES, G. A. The comparative physiological actions of dl-β-phenylisopropylamines. J. Pharmacol. & Exper. Therap. **47:** 339, 1933.

ANGELINI, C. A., AND TURLETTI, A. Sul trattamento bulgaro italiano dell'encefalite cronica. Gior. d. clin. med. **20:** 353, 1939.

ANTOLINI, A. Determinazione quantitativa degli alcaloidi totali nel decotto di radice di belladonna bulgara. Resoconto del Reparto Regina Elena. Roma, 1936.

ANTOLINI, A. Estratti concentrati da decotti vinosi e soluzioni idroalcoolicoacide di radici di belladonna bulgara. Resoconto del Reparto Regina Elena. Roma, 1936.

ANTOLINI, A. Sulle radici di atropa belladonna italiana. Resoconto del Reparto Regina Elena. Roma, 1937.

APPELRATH. Steigerung der Hautempfindlichkeit für Röntgenstrahlen bei Encephalitis lethargica. Strahlentherapie **18:** 593, 1924.

ARGHIRIS, G. Die Behandlung der Poliomyelitis (Encephalitis lethargica) und besonders deren Spätfolgen. München. med. Wchnschr. **78:** 1183, 1931.

ASKGAARD, V. Atropinbehandlung mit hohen Dosen bei Folgezuständen nach Encephalitis epidemica chronica. Acta psychiat. et neurol. **10:** 203, 1935.

ASTWAZATUROW, M. Ueber einige Kunstgriffe zur Beseitigung der extrapyramidalen Akinesen und Krämpfe. Deutsche Ztschr. f. Nervenh. **109:** 252, 1929.

AVEZZÙ, G. La scopolamina nei postumi di encefalite epidemica. Gazz. d. osp. **43:** 606, 1922.

AYMÉS, G. Essai de traitement des crises oculogyres post-encéphalitiques par les inhalations de nitrite d'amyle. Rev. d'otol. **12:** 208, 1934.

BABINSKI, J. Les syndromes parkinsoniens. Presse méd. **29:** 524, 1921.

BAILEY, A. E. Bulgarian belladonna root. Pharmaceut. J. **140:** 567, 1938.

BARKER, L. F. Diagnosis and treatment of the Parkinson-like syndromes of chronic epidemic encephalitis. Med. Clin. N. America **14:** 131, 1930.

BAUER, E., GOLSE, J., AND MARQUET, G. Le traitement du syndrome parkinsonien encéphalitique par le sulfate d'atropine à haute dose. Ann. med.-psychol. (pt. 1) **93:** 420, 1935.

BAUMANN, T. Beobachtungen über die Wirkung von Brom und Prominal bei postencephalitischen Zuständen. Schweiz. med. Wchnschr. **65:** 1188, 1935.

BAUMER, L. Der heutige Stand der Therapie der enzephalitischen Folgezustände. Psychiat.-neurol. Wchnschr. **41:** 10, 1939.

BECK, D. J. Over de zogenaande Bulgaarse kuur bij post-encephalitische afwijkingen. Psychiat. en neurol. bl. **42:** 540, 1938.

BELLONI, G. B., AND BOZZI, R. Azione del decotto bulgaro sulla catatonia umana e sperimentale. Atti d. Soc. Med.-Chir. d. Padova **13:** no. 5, 143, 1935.

BENEDEK, L., AND DE THURZÓ, J. La narcolessi genuina e la sua terapia. Riforma med. **47:** 443, 1931.

BENNET, A. E. Curare: a preventive of traumatic complications in convulsive shock therapy. Am. J. Psychiat. **97:** 1040, 1941.

BENVENUTI, M. Richerche clinico-sperimentali sulle modificazione della sindrome parkinsoniana encefalitica apportate dalla cosidetta "cura bulgara." Neopsichiatria **3:** 59, 1937.

BERINGER, K. Ueber ein neues, auf das extrapyramidal-motorische System wirkendes Alkaloid (Banisterin). Nervenarzt **1:** 265, 1928.

BERINGER, K., AND WILMANNS, K. Zur Harmin-Banisterin-Frage. Deutsche med. Wchnschr. **55:** 2081, 1929.

BIANCHINI, M. L., AND NARDI, J. Saggi di malariaterapia delle epilessie e del parkinsonismo postencefalitico. Arch. gen. di neurol. psichiat. e psicoanal. **9:** 241, 1928.

BIFULCO, C., AND EBHARDT, E. Cura dell'encefalite epidemica cronica mediante infezione ricorrente. Cervello **6:** 295, 1927.

BILLIGHEIMER, E. Die Quecksilberbehandlung bei der Encephalitis lethargica. Klin. Wchnschr. **2:** 1215, 1923.

BOHNE, O. Beobachtungen bei Encephalitis epidemica. Arch. f. Psychiat. **72:** 543, 1925.

BOSCHI, G., AND CAMPAILLA, G. Risultati della cura dei postumi dell'encefalite letargica mediante il solfato neutro di atropina. Minerva med. **26:** 903, 1935.

BOYD, E. M. On the stimulant effect of benzedrine sulphate. Proc. Soc. Exper. Biol. & Med. **37:** 127, 1937.

BOZZI, R. Osservazioni sul comportamento del sistema neuro-vegetativo negli encefalitici in cura bulgara. Policlinico (sez. prat.) **42:** 1750, 1935.

BRAGMAN, L. J. The use of stramonium in Parkinsonian states. Med. J. & Rec. **131:** 21, 1930.

BREDNOW, W. Einfluss hoher Atropindosen auf das morphologische und motorische Verhalten des Magens beim Enzephalitiker. Röntgenpraxis **7:** 183, 1935.

BREMER, F. W. Über die Unterempfindlichkeit gegenüber Atropin bei den chronisch-amyostatischen Encephalitis-Kranken. Deutsches Arch. f. klin. Med. **149:** 340, 1925.

BRISSOT, M., AND DELSUC. Parkinsonisme post-encéphalitique chez un enfant traité par la méthode de Roemer. Ann. méd.-psychol. **94:** 746, 1936.

BROEKEMA, J. C. De Behandeling van postencephalitisch Parkinsonisme. Nederl. tijdschr. v. geneesk. **82:** 3323, 1938.

BROWDER, J., AND MEYERS, R. A surgical procedure for postencephalitic tremors. Tr. Am. Neurol. A. **66:** 176, 1940.

BRÜCKL, K., AND MUSSGNUG, F. Ueber die Identität von Harmin und Banisterin. München. med. Wchnschr. **76:** 1078, 1929.

BUCY, P. C., AND CASE, T. J. Tremor: physiologic mechanism and abolition by surgical means. Arch. Neurol. & Psychiat. **41:** 721, 1939.

BUCY, P. C., AND CASE, T. J. Athetosis; surgical treatment of unilateral athetosis. Arch. Neurol. & Psychiat. **37:** 983, 1937.

BURMAN, M. S. The therapeutic use of curare and erythroidine hydrochloride for spastic and dystonic states. Arch. Neurol. & Psychiat. **41:** 307, 1939.

BURNS, M. M. The use of stramonium in the treatment of encephalitis. Psychiat. Quart. **5:** 271, 1931.

BUSSE, W. Die Behandlung der chronischen Encephalitis epidemica mit hohen Atropindosen. Arch. f. Psychiat. u. Nervenkr. **97:** 113, 1932.

CARAMAZZA, C. Le prove di funzionalità epatica nei parkinsoniani postencefalitici in rapporto alla cura con decotto di atropa belladonna. Pisani **57:** 213, 1937.

CARMICHAEL, E. A., AND GREEN, F. H. K. Parkinsonian rigidity; clinical and instrumental study of stramonium, hyoscine, and other alkoloids. Quart. J. Med. **22:** 51, 1928.

CENI, C. Sul meccanismo d'azione della cura bulgara nel parkinsonismo postencefalitico. 44 p. Bologna, 1935.

CHEVALLIER, P., SCHWOB, R., AND DURANDY. Essai de traitement de l'encéphalite léthargique par le trypanblau. Bull. et mém. Soc. méd. d. hôp. de Paris **53:** 1173, 1929.

CHIABOV, A. Pericoli delle cure con atropina nei postencefalitici durante la stagione calda. Riforma med. **52:** 56, 1936.

CHIABOV, A. Il magnesio nella terapia delle malattie mentali. Rassegna di studi psichiat. **28:** 634, 1939.

CLINQUART, E. Contribution à l'étude de la liane yagé et de son alcaloide. J. de pharmacie de Belgique **19:** 1926.

COHEN, H., AND CRAW, J. W. High hyoscine dosage in chronic encephalitis. Brit. M. J. 1937, I, 996.

COHN, H. Beitrag zur Atropinbehandlung des postencephalitischen Zustandsbildes und verwandter Erkrankungen. Klin. Wchnschr. **11:** 116, 1932.

COLOGNESE, G. Epilessia e cura Bulgara. Gior. di psichiat. e di neuropat. **64:** 210, 1936.

CONTI, A. Autosieroterapia rachidiana nel parkinsonismo post-encefalitico. Gior. di clin. med. **7:** 246, 1926.

COOPER, H. A. The treatment of oculogyric crises in chronic epidemic encephalitis. Lancet 1932, I, 290.

COSTE, M., AND DEVÈZE, M. À propos du traitement des syndromes postencéphalitique par la "cure bulgare." Bull. et mém. Soc. méd. d. hôp. de Paris **52:** 814, 1936.

CRAIG, R. N. Treatment of parkinsonian syndrome, following encephalitis, by malaria. Lancet 1927, II, 860.

DALMER, O. Weiterer Beitrag zum Identitätsbeweis der Alkoloide Harmin und Banisterin. Deutsche med. Wchnschr. **55:** 1592, 1929.

D'ANDREA, D. Un caso di postumi di encefalite epidemica osservato durante la gravidenza, il parto e il puerperio. Riv. d'Ostetrica e Ginecologia Pratica **8:** 264, 1926.

D'ARMAN, S. Postumi di encefalite letargica trattati coi raggi X. Atti Congr. ital. radiol. **5:** 144, 1924.

DAUNIC, M. Contribution à l'étude du traitement des états parkinsoniens par le datura et par l'association datura parathyroide et belladone. 58 p. Thèse de Paris, 1929.

DAVIDOFF, E. A clinical study of the effect of benzedrine therapy on self-absorbed patients. Psychiatric Quart. **10:** 652, 1936.

DAVIS, P. W., AND STEWART, W. B. Benzedrine sulphate in Parkinsonism. J. A. M. A. **110:** 1890, 1938.

DECOURT, J., AND BOCQUENTIN, A. Le traitement des syndromes parkinsoniens par l'alcaloïde du Yagé. Bull. et mém. Soc. méd. d. hôp. de Paris **53:** 1272, 1929.

DEJANOV, V. I. Resultate der Behandlung der epidemischen Encephalitis mit Pferdeserum. Abstr. in: Zentralbl. f. d. ges. Neurol. u. Psychiat. **79:** 356, 1936.

DEJANOV, V. I. Die Mangantherapie bei epidemischer Encephalitis. Abstr. in: Ann. med.-psychol. **94:** 932, 1936. Also in: Zentralbl. f. d. ges. Neurol. u. Psychiat. **78:** 225, 1935.

DELMAS-MARSALET, P. Mécanisme d'action de la bulbocapnine sur le tremblement parkinsonien. Rev. neurol. **1:** 640, 1930.

DELMAS-MARSALET, P. Essais de chirurgie physiologique dans le traitement du parkinsonisme. Rev. neurol. **63:** 550, 1935.

DETRIK, L. E., and others. On the pharmacology of phenylisopropylamine (benzedrine). J. Pharmacol. & Exper. Therap. **60:** 56, 1937.

DEVIC, A., PERRON, AND ROUGIER. Quelques essais d'un nouveau médicament des syndromes striés: l'harmine. J. de méd. de Lyon. **12:** 157, 1931.

DISERTORI, B. La cura bulgaro-italiana dell'encefalite cronica. 86 p. Roma, 1938.

DISERTORI, B. Sull'azione del solfato di betafenilisopropilamina associato alla cura di belladonna nell'encefalite letargica cronica. Policlinico (sez. prat.) **45:** 1768, 1938.

DONATELLI-CISBANI. Raffronto tra dosaggio chimico e dosaggio biologico degli alcaloidi della radice di belladonna toscana, jugoslava e bulgara. Arch. ital. Sci. farmacol. 1938.

DRESSLER, M. Benzedrin in der Behandlung des postencephalitischen Parkinsonismus. Schweiz. med. Wchnschr. **68:** 1031, 1938.

DREYFUS, G. L., AND HANAU, R. Grundsätzliches über die Verwendung des neuen Fiebermittels Saprovitan in der Neurologie. Deutsche med. Wchnschr. **52:** 1381, 1926.

DUENSING, F. Ueber die Wirkung des Apoatropins beim Menschen und seine Anwendung in der Behandlung der chronischen Encephalitis. Klin. Wchnschr. **17:** 1550, 1938.

DUENSING, F. Welche Wirkungen haben die Nebenalkaloide der Belladonnawurzel? Deutsche Ztschr. f. Nervenh. **150:** 70, 1939.

DUENSING, F., AND MEYER, L. Die Behandlung der postencephalitischen Schauanfälle mit Calcibronat. Ztschr. f. d. ges. Neurol. u. Psychiat. **162:** 136, 1938.

VON ECONOMO, C. Die Encephalitis lethargica; ihre Nachkrankheiten und ihre Behandlung. 251 p. Berlin, 1929.

EHRENBERG, L. Några ord om behahandling av postencefalitiska föejatillstand med stora atropindoser. Hygiea **94:** 785, 1932. Abstr. in: Zentralbl. f. d. ges. Neurol. u. Psychiat. **66:** 762, 1933.

EICHLER, P. Klinische und ergographische Untersuchungen über die Wirkung von Harmin und Harmalin bei Postenzephalitikern. Monatschr. f. Psychiat. u. Neurol. **74:** 152, 1929.

EMBDEN. Malariaimpfung bei postencephalitischem Parkinsonismus. Deutsche med. Wchnschr. **52:** 1214, 1926.

ENGE. Zur therapeutischen Verwendbarkeit des Neurosmon. Med. Klin. **26:** 1677, 1930.

ENGERTH, G., AND HOFF, H. Ueber das Schicksal der Patienten mit schweren Charakterveränderungen nach Encephalitis epidimeca. Deutsche med. Wchnschr. **55:** 181, 1929.

EPSTEIN, S. H., FARNHAM, R. K., AND COBB, S. The use of salicylates in the treatment of chronic epidemic encephalitis. Boston M. & S. J. **197:** 1552, 1927–28.

ESCHKE, F., AND HEMPEL, J. Zur Frage des postinfektiösen Genese des Parkinsonismus. Deutsche Ztschr. f. Nervenh. **133:** 287, 1934.

EUZIÈRE, J., PAGES, P., and others. Syndrome parkinsonien très amélioré après une fièvre typhoïde. Arch. Soc. d. sc. méd. et biol. de Montpellier. **12:** 491, 1931.

FABING, H. D. The Bulgarian belladonna treatment of postencephalitic Parkinsonian syndrome. Ohio State M. J. **35:** 1195, 1939.

FASTING, G. Disappearance of creatinuria after lactic acid therapy. New Orleans M. & S. J. **87:** 467, 1935.

FAURE-BEAULIEU, M., AND CORD, M. L'harmine, nouvelle médication anti-parkinsonienne. Rev. méd. franç. **12:** 445, 1931.

FAWCITT, R. Treatment of encephalitis lethargica associated with Parkinsonism by ultra-violet rays. Brit. M. J. 1927, I, 422.

FEHSENMEIER, H. Klinische Untersuchungen über das Verhalten des Magen-Darmkanals bei mit Atropin behandelten Enzephalitikern. München. med. Wchnschr. **82:** 1723, 1935.

FERRANNINI, L. Contributo clinico alla cura bulgaro dei postumi di encefalite letargica. Med. nuova **26:** 230, 1935.

FERRANDO, E. Sulla cura atropinica del parkinsonismo postencefalitico. Note e riv. d. psichiat. **65:** 441, 1936.

LE FÈVRE DE ARRIC, M. Sur le traitement de l'encéphalite épidémique et de ses séquelles par le virus-vaccin. Le Scalpel **78:** 396, 1925.

FINKELMAN, I., AND SHAPIRO, L. B. Benzedrine sulphate and atropine in treatment of chronic encephalitis. J. A. M. A. **109:** 344, 1937.

FISCHER, A. Untersuchungen über die Wirkung des Alkaloides Harmin bei postenzephalitischen Zuständen. München. med. Wchnschr. **76:** 451, 1929.

FLECK, U. Über Erfahrungen mit der Behandlung chronischer Enzephalitiker auf der Göttinger Encephalitisstation. Deutsche med. Wchnschr. **59:** 55, 1933.

FLECK, U., AND RUSTIGE, E. Über den Verlauf der chronischen Encephalitis epidemica. Arch. f. Psychiat. **97:** 101, 1932.

FLEISCHHACKER, H. Ueber den Einfluss des Bulbocapninum hydrochloricum auf verschiedene Hyperkinesen. Deutsche med. Wchnschr. **52:** 352, 1926.

FLURY, F. Uber Harmin bzw. Banisterin. München. med. Wchnschr. **76:** 1172, 1929.

FRAENKEL, M. Die Beeinflussung des übermässigen Speichelflusses bei Encephalitis lethargica chronica durch temporäre Parotisausschaltung mittels Roentgenstrahlen. Deutsche med. Wchnschr. **49:** 613, 1923.

FRANK, H., AND SCHLESINGER, O. Klinische Erfahrungen bei der Behandlung der postencephalitischen Erscheinungen mit Harmin. Klin. Wchnschr. **9:** 1864, 1930.

FROMENT, J. Onirisme postencéphalitique séquellaire amélioré par l'insuline. Rev. neurol. **37:** 1162, 1930.

FROMENT, J. Dédoublement de la personalité et amnésie profonde.... Compt. rend. Cong. d. médecins alién. et neurol. **38:** 309, 1934.

FROMENT, J., BADINAND, A., AND DUVAL, M. L'insuline, en atténuant les effets second du Parkinsonisme rétablit le taux, parfois abaissé, de la réserve alcaline. Arch. internat. de Neurol. **22:** 197, 1930.

FUCHS, A. Säure-Diät-Therapie der chronischen Encephalitis. Allg. Ztschr. f. Psychiat. **93:** 115, 1930.

FURBURY, J. Vaccin de Levaditi et Parkinsonisme post-encéphalitique. 63 p. Thèse de Toulouse, 1926.

GAMARNIK, I. J. Behandlung des postencephalitischen Parkinsonismus mit Kalium hypermanganicum. Abstr. in Zentralbl. f. d. ges. Neurol. u. Psychiat. **75:** 68, 1935.

GAMBLE, C. J., PEPPER, O. H., AND MULLER, G. P. Postencephalitic tic of diaphragma. J. A. M. A. **85:** 1485, 1925.

GAMPER, E. Paralysis agitans. In: Handbuch der Neurologie. XVI, 757. Berlin, 1936.

GANDELLINI, A. Sul nuovo indirizzo terapeutico dei postumi della encefalite letargica. Gazz. d. osp. **59:** 421, 1938.

GANGL, P., AND LUCKSCH, F. C Vitamin und Encephalitis epidemica. Klin. Wchnschr. **18:** 1193, 1939.

GAUSEBECK, H. Versuche mit Harmin hydrochlor. bei Parkinsonismus. Psychiat.-neurol. Wchnschr. **31:** 386, 1929.

GAYLE, R. F., JR. The treatment of infections of the central nervous system by forced spinal drainage. Virginia M. Month. **61:** 228, 1934.

GAYLE, R. F., JR. Treatment of parkinsonism with preparation of belladonna root. Virginia M. Month. **66:** 707, 1939.

GAYLE, R. F., JR., AND WILLIAMS, J. N. The symptomatic treatment of the parkinsonian syndrome with cobra venom. South. M. J. **31:** 188, 1938.

GILLESPIE, I. A. Treatment of post-encephalitis. J. Ment. Sc. **74:** 410, 1928.

GLOWINSKI, B. I. Le traitement de la maladie de Parkinson par le datura injectable. 47 p. Thèse de Paris, 1933.

GOLDBERG, S. A. Roentgen therapy in cases of encephalitis. Arch. Neurol. & Psychiat. **37:** 446, 1937.

GOUREVITSCH, I. S. Ephedrinbehandlung der Schauanfälle bei postencephalitischem Parkinsonismus. Abstr. in: Zentralbl. f. d. ges. Neurol. u. Psychiat. **86:** 544, 1937.

GOWLLAND, E. Hyoscine in Parkinsonism. Brit. M. J. 1935, II, 877.

GREEN, F. H. K. Two cases of post-encephalitic Parkinsonism: To illustrate the results of treatment by hyoscine and by stramonium. Proc. Roy. Soc. Med. **21:** 321, 1927–28.

GREWEL, F. Atropinebehandeling bij post-encephalitisch Parkinsonisme. Nederl. tijdschr. v. geneesk. **82:** 1569, 1938.

GUNN, J. A. A note on banisterine or harmine. Lancet 1929, I, 769.

GUNN, J. A. Some pharmacological actions of banisterine (harmine). Lancet 1929, I, 1140.

GUNN, J. A., AND MACKEITH, R. C. The pharmacological actions of harmol. Quart. J. Pharm. & Pharmacol. **4:** 33, 1931.

GUNN, J. A., AND SIMONART, A. J. L. The pharmacological actions of harmalol. Quart. J. Pharm. & Pharmacol. **3:** 218, 1930.

HAGSTRÖM, O. Nagra erfarenheter av behandlingen av encephalitska fojdtillstanden ligti Roemer. Svenska läk.-tidning. **31:** 369, 1934. Abstr. in: Zentralbl. f. d. ges. Neurol. u. Psychiatr. **73:** 186, 1934.

HALL, A. J. Post-encephalitic Parkinsonism, with some remarks on the results of treatment by belladonna. Brit. M. J. 1926, I, 127.

HALL, A. J. Drugs in post-encephalitic Parkinsonism. Lancet 1934, I, 595.

HALL, A. J. The results of high atropine dosage in chronic epidemic encephalitis. Brit. M. J. 1937, II, 795.

HALL, G. W. Narcolepsy. Med. Clin. N. America **17:** 1483, 1934.

HALPERN, L. Der Wirkungsmechanismus des Harmins und die Pathophysiologie der Parkinsonschen Krankheit. Deutsche med. Wchnschr. **56:** 651, 1930.

HALPERN, L. Ueber die Harminwirkung im Selbstversuch. Deutsche med. Wchnschr. **56:** 1252, 1930.

HARROWER, G., AND GHOSH, K. C. Bilateral first thoracic ganglionectomy in two cases of Parkinson's syndrome. Brit. M. J. 1933, II, 722.

HASSLER, R. Zur pathologischen Anatomie des senilen und des parkinsonistischen Tremor. J. f. Psychol. u. Neurol. **49:** 193, 1939.

HECHLER, H. Erfahrungen mit der "Bulgarischen Kur" (Homburg 680). München. med. Wchnschr. **86:** 1264, 1939.

HENRIKSEN, R. H. Bulgarian belladonna. Pharmaceutical J. **140:** 240, 1938.

HENRIKSEN, R. H. Bulgarian belladonna. Pharmaceutical J. **141:** 522, 1938.

HERRMANN, G. Affektiver Tonusverlust (Lachschlag Oppenheims) nach Encephalitis epidemica und seine Beeinflussung durch Strychnin. Med. Klin. **24:** 854, 1928.

HERRMANN, G., AND WOTKE, E. Die Beeinflussung des Tremors bei Encephalopathia postgripposa durch Nikotin. Med. Klin. **21:** 1842, 1925.

HERSCHMANN, H. [Erfahrungen in der Wiener Psychiatrischen Universitätsklinik mit der Malariatherapie]. Verhandl. d. deutsch. Gesellsch. f. inn. Med. 1923, 76.

HESS, L., AND FALTISCHEK, J. Ueber Innervationsstörungen des Magens bei Parkinsonismus. Wien. med Wchnschr. **40:** 409, 457, 1927.

HILL, D. Bulgarian treatment of post-encephalitic Parkinsonism. Lancet 1938, II, 1048.

HILL, T. R. Juvenile behaviour disorders in epidemic encephalitis; their treatment by bulbocapnine. Lancet 1929, I, 968.

HILL, T. R., AND WORSTER-DROUGHT, C. Observations on harmine in the treatment of chronic epidemic encephalitis. Lancet 1929, II, 647.

HOEDEMAKER, E. D., AND BURNS, M. A. The effect of stramonium in Parkinsonism. Arch. Neurol. & Psychiat. **24:** 869, 1930.

HÖGLUND, G., AND SJÖGREN, V. H. Traitement des formes chroniques de l'encéphalite léthargique par la fièvre récurrente. Acta psychiat. et neurol. **6:** 397, 1931.

HÖNIG, E. Über Behebung von Schluckstörungen bei bulbären Läsionen mit den Stossübungen. Nervenarzt **10:** 193, 1937.

HÖNIG, E. Über Behebung von bulbären Schluckstörungen (Nachtrag). Nervenarzt **13:** 9, 1940.

HOFF, H. Uebersicht der therapeutischen Versuche bei der Encephalitis lethargica auf der Klinik vom 1 Jänner 1916 bis 30 Mai 1923. Wien. klin. Wchnschr. **36:** 899, 1923.

HOHMANN, L. B. The treatment of post-encephalitic Parkinson syndrome with hyoscin hydrobromide, with a note on the mental attitude in this syndrome and report of 18 cases. Bull. Johns Hopkins Hosp. **35:** 335, 1924.

HUNTER, J. I. The influence of the sympathetic nervous system in the genesis of rigidity of striated muscle in spastic paralysis. Surg. Gynec. Obst. **39:** 721, 1924.

INGEBRIGTSEN, B. Surgical treatment of post-encephalitic involuntary movements of the tongue. Acta psychiat. et neurol. **12:** 55, 1937.

INGRAM, W. R., AND RANSON, S. W. Bulbocapnine; effect on animals with lesions of the central nervous system. Arch. Neurol. & Psychiat. **31:** 987, 1934.

JACOBI, E. Harminbehandlung bei chronischer Enzephalitis. München. med. Wchnschr. **77:** 929, 1930.

JACOBSON, A. L., AND EPPLEN, F. Later results in the use of stramonium in postencephalitic syndrome. Ann. Int. Med. **4:** 145, 1930.

JAFFÉ, H. N. Encephalitis lethargica associated with Parkinsonism treated by ultra-violet rays. Brit. M. J. 1927, II, 1219.

JENKINS, R. L., AND ROWLEY, C. C. Bulbocapnine in the treatment of behavior disorders such as occur in chronic epidemic encephalitis. J. Nerv. & Ment. Dis. **84:** 507, 1936.

JEWETT, S. P., and others. High dosage atropine therapy in chronic encephalitic Parkinsonism. Am. J. M. Sc. **195:** 809, 1938.

JOLIFFE, N. Clinical aspects of vitamin B deficiences. Minnesota Med. **23:** 542, 1940.

JOLIFFE, N. Effects of vitamin B_6 in paralysis agitans. Tr. Am. Neurol. A. **66:** 54, 1940.

JOLIFFE, N. Further results of vitamin B_6 therapy in paralysis agitans. Paper read at meeting of Section on Neurology and Psychiatry, New York Academy of Medicine, December 10, 1940.

de Jong, H. Experimenteele en clinische catatonie. Nederl. tijdschr. v. geneesk. **73:** 640, 1929.

de Jong, H., and Herman, W. The action of bulbocapnine in three cases of paralysis agitans and one case of tremor of paralysis agitans type. . . . Arch. Neurol. & Psychiat. **16:** 55, 1926.

de Jong, H., and Schaltenbrand, G. Further clinical investigations with bulbocapnine. Neurotherapie **7:** 1, 1925.

Juster, E. Traitement de la rigidité parkinsonienne par la stramoine. Rev. neurol. **32:** 218, 1925.

Juster, E. Au sujet de l'administration du datura stramonium chez les parkinsoniens. Presse méd. **35:** 329, 1927.

Juster, E., and Huerre, R. Traitement des états parkinsoniens par la stramoine. Bull. gén. de thérap. **177:** 133, 1926.

Kairiukschtis, V., and Kutorga, V. Versuche die Muskelrigidität beim Parkinsonismus durch Injektion von Kurare zu beseitigen. München. med. Wchnschr. **74:** 537, 1927.

Katona, T. Die Behandlung des encephalitischen Parkinsonismus. Abstr. in: Zentralbl. f. d. ges. Neurol. u. Psychiat. **44:** 336, 1926.

Kauders, O., and Oesterreicher, W. Ueber die Wirksamkeit der sogenannten bulgarischen Kur beim Parkinsonismus im Vergleiche zur Behandlung mit hohen Atropindosen. Wien. klin. Wchnschr. **49:** 1548, 1936.

Kidd, H. A. Bilateral superior thoracic ganglion neurectomy in parkinsonism. Brit. M. J. 1933, I, 99.

Kiss, N., and Szirmák, B. Neue Röntgenbestrahlungsmethode der Parkinson-Krankheit. Röntgenpraxis **6:** 746, 1934.

Klaue, R. Parkinsonsche Krankheit (Paralysis agitans) und postencephalitischer Parkinsonismus. Arch. f. Psychiat. **111:** 251, 1940.

Kleemann, A. Mitteilung zur Therapie der chronischen Encephalitis. Deutsche Ztschr. f. Nervenh. **111:** 299, 1929.

Koepchen, A. Zur Differentialdiagnose der Muskelstarre bei Parkinsonscher Krankheit und Parkinsonismus. Deutsche med. Wchnschr. **48:** 1071, 1922.

Kraus, F. Eine neue Methode der Hyperämiebehandlung chronischer Gehirn- und Rückenmarkserkrankungen durch Diathermie. Med. Klin. **25:** 1929, 1929.

Krause, P. Röntgentherapeutische Versuche bei Kranken mit Enzephalitis und Folgezuständen. Strahlentherapie **44:** 33, 1932.

Kürbitz, W. Therapeutische Erfahrungen bei chronischen Enzephalitikern. Allg. Ztschr. f. Psychiat. **89:** 390, 1928.

Kürbitz, W., and Lange, W. Impfmalaria bei chronischer Encephalitis epidemica. Psychiat.-neurol. Wchnschr. **31:** 67, 1929.

LADOS, J. Contribution à l'étude du traitement du syndrome parkinsonien post-encéphalitique par l'aminoxyde de Scopolamine (Génoscopolamine). 109 p. Thèse de Lyon, 1927.

LAIGNEL-LAVASTINE, AND STERNE, J. Le traitement par le bleu de trypane des parkinsoniens d'origine encéphalitique. Bull. et mém. Soc. méd. d. hôp. de Paris **48:** 689, 1932.

LAIGNEL-LAVASTINE, AND VALENCE, R. Résultats d'un an de traitement des syndromes parkinsoniens par le datura stramonium. Bull. et mém. Soc. méd. d. hôp. de Paris **50:** 921, 1926.

LAMPL, O. Zur Therapie der encephalitischen Folgezustände. Med. Klin. **24:** 136, 1928.

LAMPL, O. Weitere Beiträge zur symptomatischen Therapie der chronischen Encephalitis. Med. Klin. **25:** 1353, 1929.

LANGE, W., AND SCHNEIDER, W. Ergebnisse der Röntgenbestrahlung bei chronischer Encephalitis epidemica. Psychiat.-neurol. Wchnschr. **34:** 7, 1932.

LEINER, J. H., AND KAUFMAN, M. R. Bulbocapnine in diseases manifesting dyskinesia; clinical and therapeutic observations in 19 cases divided into groups. Arch. Neurol. & Psychiat. **20:** 1269, 1928.

LEMOINE, G. Resection des rameaux communicants lombaires pour syndrome parkinsonien encéphalitique. Le Scalpel **79:** 721, 1926.

LEMOS, M. Actions de la scopolamine sur le clonus et la réflectivité en général dans un cas de syndrome parkinsonien postencéphalitique prolongé. Rev. neurol. **30:** II, 424, 1923.

LERICHE, R. De l'intervention chirurgicale dans la maladie de Parkinson. Lyon chirurg. **7:** 287, 1921.

LEQUIN, A. Traitement des formes parkinsoniennes de l'encéphalite épidémique par les injections intraveineuses de salicylate de soude glucosé. 79 p. Thèse de Paris, 1928.

LEREBOULLET, J. Le traitement belladonné des syndromes parkinsoniens. Paris méd. **28:** 69, 1938.

LEVI-BIANCHINI, M. Osservazioni sulla "cura bulgara". . . . Arch. gen. di neurol. psichiat. e psicoanal. **18:** 35, 1937.

LEWENSTEIN, H. Die Behandlung der Folgezustände der Encephalitis epidemica mit hohen Atropindosen. Deutsche med. Wchnschr. **57:** 1014, 1931.

LEWENSTEIN, H. Die Behandlung der Encephalitis epidemica und ihrer Folgezustände mit hohen Atropindosen. Arch. f. Psychiat. u. Nervenh. **94:** 198, 1931.

LEWIN, L. Banisteria Caapi, ein neues Rauschgift und Heilmittel. Beitr. zur Giftkunde, Heft 3. Berlin, 1929.

LEWIN, L., AND SCHUSTER, P. Ergebnisse von Banisterinversuchen an Nervenkranken, Med. Klin. **25:** 562, 1929.

LISAK, A. Die Atropinbehandlung des postenzephalitischen Parkinsonismus. Schweiz. med. Wchnschr. **13:** 672, 1932.

LOREY, A. AND SCHALTENBRAND, G. Pachymeningitis nach Röntgenbestrahlung? Strahlentherapie **44:** 747, 1932.

LUST, F. Ueber die Beeinflussung der postenzephalitischen Schlafstörung durch temperatursteigernde Mittel. Deutsche med. Wchnschr. **47:** 1545, 1921.

MACHANSKY, F. I. Traitement chirurgical des mouvements involontaires des extrémités appliqué au parkinsonisme postencéphalitique. J. de chir. **46:** 877, 1935.

MAIDAN-MAIDANSKY, E. M. [Potassium permanganate for treating postencephalitic paralysis agitans] Mosk. med. j. **8:** no. 2, 30, 1928. Abstr. in: Zentrabl. f. d. ges. Neurol. u. Psychiat. **50:** 156, 1928.

MAIER, H. W. Zur Behandlung der parkinsonistischen Folgezustände nach Encephalitis epidemica. Schweiz. med. Wchnschr. **68:** 1354, 1938.

MAIN, T. F. Post-traumatic Parkinsonism and the effect of atropine. Brit. M. J. 1938, I, 170.

MALMROS, R. Om Atropinbehandling af den postencephalitiske Parkinsonisme. Hospitalstid. **79:** 865, 1936. Abstr. in: Zentralbl. f. d. ges. Neurol. u. Psychiat. **84:** 104, 1937.

MARBURG, O., AND SGALITZER, M. Die Röntgenbehandlung der Nervenkrankheiten. Wien, 1930.

MARCUS, H., KLING, C., AND HÖGLUND, G. Le traitement de l'encéphalite épidémique chronique par l'infection récurrente. Compt. rend. Soc. de biol. **95:** 749, 1926.

MARGUGLIO, D., AND TRIPI, G. Gli estratti fluidi di radici di belladonna italiana nella cura delle syndromi parkinsoniane postencefalitiche. Pisani **57:** 281, 1937.

MARIE, A., AND POINCLOUX, P. Essai de vaccino-thérapie intrarachidienne des séquelles de l'encéphalite épidémique avec du virus fixe encéphalitique. Bull. Acad. de méd., Paris **91:** 322, 1924.

MARIE, A., POINCLOUX, P., AND CODET, H. Traitement d'un cas de parkinsonisme post-encéphalitique par injection intra-rachidienne de virus vaccin encéphalitique. Encéphale **19:** 421, 1924.

MARINESCO, G., AND FAÇON, E. L'atropine à doses progressives et fortes dans le traitement des troubles postencéphalitiques. Bull. Acad. de méd., Paris **115:** 493, 1936.

MARINESCO, G., AND FAÇON, E. Quelques remarques sur la "cure bulgare" des troubles postencéphalitiques. Bull. et mém. Soc. méd. d. hôp. de Paris **52:** 670, 1936.

Marinesco, G., Kreindler, A., and Façon, E. Action de l'injection intrarachidienne de novocaine sur la rigidité parkinsonienne. Compt. rend. Soc. de biol. **105:** 916, 1930.

Marinesco, G., Kreindler, A., and Scheim, A. Klinische und experimentelle Beiträge zur Pharmakologie des Harmins. Arch. f. exper. Path. u. Pharmakol. **154:** 301, 1930.

Marinesco, G., Sager, O., and Kreindler, A. Mécanisme de l'action thérapeutique de la scopolamine chez les parkinsoniens postencéphalitiques. Compt. rend. Soc. de biol. **98:** 1322, 1928.

Marx, E. Zur Symptomatologie und Therapie der chronischen Encephalitis lethargica. München. med. Wchnschr. **74:** 1916, 1927.

Más de Ayala, I. Tratamiento por el "Treponema hispanicum" de afecciones mentales y neurológicas. Resultados obtenidos en 200 enfermos tratados. An. de Fac. de med., Montevideo **14:** 605 (French summary 631), 1929. Abstr. in: Zentralbl. f. d. ges. Neurol. u. Psychiat. **55:** 66, 1930.

di Mattei, P. Sulla cosidetta "cura bulgara" dei postumi di encefalite epidemica. Policlinico (sez. prat.) **42:** 501, 1935.

Matthews, R. A. Symptomatic treatment of chronic encephalitis with benzedrine sulphate. Am. J. M. Sc. **195:** 448, 1938.

Mattioli-Foggia, C. Sull trattamento del parkinsonismo postencefalitico con un metodo derivato dalla cosidetta cura bulgara. Note Psychiat. **66:** 113, 1937.

McCartan, W. Trypan-blue intravenously in postencephalitic Parkinsonism. Lancet 1934, II, 601.

McCowan, P. K., and Cook, L. C. Chronic epidemic encephalitis; treatment by induced malaria. Lancet 1927, II, 861.

McCowan, P. K., and Harris, J. S. Chronic epidemic encephalitis; scopolamine therapy. J. Ment. Sc. **73:** 40, 1927.

Meco, O. La remission della sintomatologia demenziale negli encefalitici sottoposti alla cura bulgara. Riv. di pat. nerv. e ment. **50:** 75, 1937.

Meco, O. Sindrome delirante-allucinatoria provocabile negli encefalitici sottoposti "cura bulgara." Cervello **16:** 191, 1937.

Medea, E. Nel trattamento del parkinsonismo encefalitico, l'introduzione d'aria nei ventricoli cerebrali dà veramente qualche risultato? Riv. sper. di freniat. **54:** 904, 1931.

Medea, E. A proposito del cosidetto trattamento bulgaro del parkinsonismo postencefalitico. Milano, 1936.

Meerloo, A. M. Therapeutische aanteekeningen enkelzijdig en dubbelzijdig parkinsonisme. Psychiat. en neurol. **39:** 636, 1935.

MEERLOO, A. M. Die paradoxe und wechselnde Wirkung der Barbitursäurederivate. (Ihr. Verhalten bei Encephalopathien). Ztschr. f. d. ges. Neurol. u. Psychiat. **143:** 722, 1932–33.

MELLA, H. Bulbocapnin: Its use in the treatment of tremor and in the experimental production of basal ganglion symptomatology. Arch. Neurol. & Psychiat. **15:** 325, 1926.

MENARD, O. J., AND HURXTHAL, L. M. Results of the use of stramonium datura in Parkinson's disease. . . . New England J. Med. **205:** 759, 1931.

MEYER, E. Die Beeinflussung der Bewegungsstörungen bei der Encephalitis lethargica durch rhythmische Gefühle. München. med. Wchnschr. **50:** 139, 1923.

MEYER, O. Zur Behandlung der Encephalitis lethargica. Zentralbl. f. inn. Med. **59:** 705, 1938.

MODONESI, C. Cura atropinica e cura di belladonna nel parkinsonismo da encefalite cronica. Note e riv. di psichiat. **65:** 21, 1936.

MOLL, H. The treatment of post-encephalitic Parkinsonism by nicotine. Brit. M. J. 1926, I, 1079.

MOORE, R. Treatment of encephalitis. J. A. M. A. **81:** 928, 1923.

MYERSON, A. The physiological and psychological effects of benzedrine. J. Nerv. & Ment. Dis. **85:** 202, 1937.

MYERSON, A., AND BERLIN, D. D. Case of postencephalitic Parkinson's disease treated by total thyroidectomy. New England J. Med. **210:** 1205, 1934.

NANNIZZI, A. Sulla possibilità della raccolta della belladonna spontanea e della sua coltivazione. . . . Sienna, 1937.

NANNIZZI, A. La belladonna nella cura del parkinsonismo postencefalitico. Siena, 1938.

NATALI, G., AND CAMPANACCI. La cura dell'encefalite epidemica con iniezioni endovenose di soluzione di Pregl. Sperimentale **76:** 419, 1922.

NATHANSON, M. H. The central action of beta-aminopropylbenzene (benzedrine). J. A. M. A. **108:** 528, 1937.

NAUMOW, F. Subarachnoidale Eigenbluteinführung bei Epilepsie und postencephalitischem Parkinsonismus. Abstr. in: Zentralbl. f. d. ges. Neurol. u. Psychiat. **80:** 88, 1936.

NEAL, J. B. Encephalitis: a Clinical Study. 563 p. New York, 1942.

NEAL, J. B. Recent advances in the treatment of epidemic encephalitis. New York State J. Med. **34:** 707, 1934.

NEAL, J. B. Bulgarian belladonna treatment of chronic encephalitis. New York State J. Med. **39:** 1875, 1939.

NEAL, J. B., AND BENTLEY, J. A. Treatment of epidemic encephalitis. Arch. Neurol. & Psychiat. **28**: 897, 1932.

NEUWAHL, F. J. Treatment of Parkinsonism with Bulgarian belladonna. Lancet 1939, I, 619.

NEUWAHL, F. J., AND FENWICK, C. C. Bulgarian treatment of post-encephalitic Parkinsonism. Lancet 1937, II, 619.

NEYMANN, C. A. Artificial fever produced by physical means; its development and application. 294 p. Springfield, 1938.

NIELSEN, O. J. Atropinbehandlingen af den postencephalitiske Parkinsonisme. Hospitalstid. **78**: 806, 1935. Abstr. in: Brit. M. J. 1935, II, 92.

NIKOLOFF, P. Über die sogenannte "cura bulgara" der Folgezustände der Encephalitis epidemica. Fortschr. d. Therap. **12**: 412, 1936.

NOTO, G. G. Metodo di Roemer e "cura bulgara" nel parkinsonismo postencefalitico. Rassegna di studi psichiat. **25**: 969 (English summary 979), 1936.

NUVOLI, U. La radioterapia dell'encefalite epidemica nel suo stadio acuto. Policlinico (sez. med.) **36**: 177, 1929.

OESTERREICHER, W. Zungentics bei postenphalitischem Parkinsonismus mit hohen Atropindosen behandelt. Wien. med. Klin. **33**: 318, 1937.

OLSEN, A. Behandlung der chronischen Encephalitis mit intravenösen Jodnatriumeinspritzungen. Abstr. in: Zentralbl. f. d. ges. Neurol. u. Psychiat. **81**: 205, 1936.

D'ORMEA, A., AND BROGGI, E. La "cura bulgara" nei postumi nervosi e psichichi della encefalite letargica. Rassegna di studi psichiat. **25**: 125, 1936.

ORNSTEIN, I., AND ORESTIANU, I. Sur le traitement mercuriel dans le parkinsonisme postencéphalitique. Bull. Soc. roum. neurol. **4**: no. 4, 26, 1930. Abstr. in: Zentralbl. f. d. ges. Neurol. u. Psychiat. **58**: 803, 1930–31.

OTIS, W. J. Chronic encephalitis; stramonium treatment. South. M. J. **24**: 314, 1931.

PAASCHE, K. Zur Frage der Therapie bei postencephalitischen Krankheitsformen. Allg. Ztschr. f. Psychiat. **83**: 114, 1925.

PANEGROSSI, G. Sulla così detta "cura bulgara" del parkinsonismo postencefalitico. Policlinico (sez. prat.) **42**: 506, 1935.

PANEGROSSI, G. Sulle recenti acquisizioni nella cura del parkinsonismo encefalitico. Policlinico (sez. prat.) **42**: 1487, 1935.

PANSDORF, H., AND TRAUTMANN, E. Ueber die entzündungswidrige Bestrahlung des Gehirns. Röntgenpraxis **2**: 393, 1930.

PASS, K. E. Die verschiedenen Arten der Enzephalitis. . . . Therap. d. Gegenw. **80:** 401, 1939.

PATRY, F. L. The diagnosis and treatment of postencephalitic Parkinsonism, with case report. J. Nerv. & Ment. Dis. **69:** 617, 1929.

PAULIAN, D. Sur le traitement de l'encéphalite épidémique et ses séquelles, le parkinsonisme. Rev. neurol. **32:** 86, 1925.

PERKINS, O. C. Chronic encephalitis; care and treatment of patients found in state and municipal hospitals. New York State J. Med. **36:** 255, 1936.

PESCI, E. L'antimonio nell'encefalite epidemica. Patologica **16:** no. 363 23, 1924. Abstr. in: Zentralbl. f. d. ges. Neurol. u. Psychiat. **36,** 441, 1924.

PETTE, H. Ueber endolumbale Eigenserumtherapie bei Folgezuständen von epidemischen Enzephalitis. München. med. Wchnschr. **73:** 1025, 1926.

PFEILER, R. Behandlung der chronischen Encephalitis epidemica mit Bellafolin. Med. Klin. **29:** 1623, 1933.

PIDONE. La radioterapia nei postumi di encefalite letargica. Radiol. med. **11:** 525, 1924.

PINÉAS, H. Klinische Beobachtungen über die Wirkung von Harmin. Deutsche med. Wchnschr. **55:** 910, 1929.

PITICARIN, J. Die Behandlung der Myoklonien und des Parkinsonschen Symptomenkomplexes nach Encephalitis epidemica mit intravenösen Injektionen von eigner Lumbalflüssigkeit. Wien. klin. Wchnschr. **35:** 441, 1922.

PODESTÀ, V. La radioterapia delle malattie sistematiche del sistema nervoso centrale specialamente in rapporto ai postumi di encefalite letargica. Radiol. med. **11:** 58, 1924.

POLKOVNIKOVA, E., AND BOURAČEVSKIJ, J. [Über die Toleranz gegenüber Atropin beim Parkinsonismus]. Med.-biol. zhur. **4:** 119 (French summary 126), 1928. Abstr. in: Zentralbl. f. d. ges. Neurol. u. Psychiat. **52:** 824, 1929.

POLLET, H. L. J. Contribution à l'étude du bleu de trypane. 38 p. Thèse de Paris, 1932.

POLLOK, L. J., AND DAVIS, L. Muscle tone in Parkinsonian states. Tr. Am. Neurol. A. **55:** 171, 1929.

POLONOVSKI, M. Sur les génalcaloïdes. Compt. rend. Soc. de biol. **94:** 145, 1926.

POLONOVSKI, M., AND MAX. Sur les aminoxydes des alcaloïdes du groupe du tropane. Compt. rend. Acad. Sc. **180:** 1755, 1925.

POUPPIRT, P. S. Treatment of Parkinson's syndrome with fever produced by baths. California & West. Med. **31:** 192, 1929.

PRINZMETAL, M., AND BLOOMBERG, W. The use of benzedrine for the treatment of narcolepsy. J. A. M. A. **105:** 2051, 1935.

PROPPER, N. [Treatment of parkinsonism with solutions of sodium cacodylate and Datura stramonium]. Zhur. nevropat. i psikhiat. **23,** no. 3: 91, 1930. Abstr. in: Zentralbl. f. d. ges. Neurol. u. Psychiat. **59:** 233, 1931.

PROPPER, N., AND DARKSHEVITCH, V. L. [Oxytherapy in Parkinson's disease]. Zhur. nevropat. i psikhiat. **23:** no. 4, 104, 1930. Abstr. in: Zentralbl. f. d. ges. Neurol. u. Psychiat. **59:** 602, 1931.

PUTNAM, T. J. Treatment of athetosis and dystonia by section of extrapyramidal motor tracts. Arch. Neurol. & Psychiat. **29:** 504, 1933.

PUTNAM, T. J. Relief from unilateral paralysis agitans by section of the pyramidal tract. Arch. Neurol. & Psychiat. **40:** 1049, 1938.

RADOVICI, A. L'action de l'atropine sur l'hypertonie post-encéphalitique; parkinsonisme, tremblements. . . . Presse méd. **33:** 555, 1925.

REES, C. E. Observations following sympathetic ganglionectomy in cases of post-encephalitic Parkinsonian syndrome. Am. J. Surg. **21:** 411, 1933.

RENAUD, M. Echec d'une vaccination non spécifique dans le syndrome parkinsonien post-encéphalitique. Bull. et mém. Soc. d. hôp. de Paris **48:** 1479, 1924.

RETAN, G. M. Some clinical applications of forced drainage to various infections in inflammatory conditions in the central nervous system. Arch. Neurol. & Psychiat. **29:** 404, 1933.

REZNIKOFF, L. Effect of benzedrine sulfate in treatment of psychosis with postencephalitic Parkinsonism. Arch. Neurol. & Psychiat. **42:** 112, 1939.

RIGGS, C. E. Therapy of post-encephalitic Parkinson syndrome, two cases. Minnesota Med. **10:** 135, 1927.

RIZZATI, E., AND MORENO, G. Cordotomia laterale posteriore nella cura delle ipertonie estrapiramidali postencefalitiche. Schizofrenie **5:** 117, 1936.

ROCH, M. M., AND KATZENELBOGEN. Traitement des formes évolutives chroniques de l'encéphalite épidémique, par les injections intrarachidiennes de caséine. Schweiz. med. Wchnschr. **54:** 834, 1924.

ROEMER, C. Die Atropinbehandlung der encephalitischen Folgezustände. Ztschr. f. d. ges. Neurol. u. Psychiat. **132:** 724, 1931.

ROQUES, F. Epidemic encephalitis in association with pregnancy, labour and puerperium; review and report of 21 cases. Obst. & Gynæc. Brit. Emp. **35:** 1, 1928.

ROSENBERGER, A. Klinische Erfahrungen über die Wirkung des Harmins bei postencephalitischem Parkinsonismus. Wien. klin. Wchnschr. **43:** 207, 1930.

ROSENBUND, L. Beeinflussung des senilen Tremors und anderer Tremorarten durch Salicylsäure. Med. Klin. **25:** 563, 1929.

ROSENOW, E. C. Specific serum treatment of epidemic encephalitis. J. A. M. A. **80:** 1583, 1923.

ROSENTHAL, C. Zur Therapie der Encephalitis epidemica. Klin. Wchnschr. **5:** 1105, 1926.

ROSIN, H. Ueber die Behandlung des Parkinsonismus mit Striaphorin. Deutsche med. Wchnschr. **56:** 1046, 1930.

ROYLE, N. D. The treatment of spastic paralysis by sympathetic ramisection. Surg. Gynec. & Obstet. **39:** 701, 1924.

ROYLE, N. D. Clinical results following operation of sympathetic ramisection. Canad. M. A. J. **24:** 229, 1931.

RUBINO, A. La sieroreazione di Weltmann e colesterinemia. Bull. Soc. med. chir. Catania 4, 1936.

RUSSETZKI, J. J. [Ueber den Einfluss von Chlorcalcium und Chlormagnesium auf den Muskeltonus des Parkinsonikern]. Med.-biol. zhur. **4:** 84 (French summary 88), 1928. Abstr. in: Zentralbl. f. d. ges. Neurol. u. Psychiat. **52:** 216, 1929.

RUSTIGE, E. Versuche mit Harmin bei Metenzephalitikern. Deutsche med. Wchnschr. **55:** 613, 1929.

SǍFÁR, K., AND SPITZMÜLLER, W. Über Behandlung von schwerem Lidkrampf mit Elektrokoagulation. Klin. Wchnschr. **11:** 405, 1932.

SAHLGREN, E. Bemerkenswerte schädliche Wirkungen bei Atropinbehandlung. Deutsche Ztschr. f. Nervenh. **143:** 283, 1937.

SANTANGELO, G. Su la cura del Parkinsonismo post-encefalitico. Cervello **2:** 321, 1923.

SAUTER, E. Zum Schicksal der Encephalitiker. Schweiz. med. Wchnschr. **64:** 464, 1934.

SCHALTENBRAND, G. Ueber die Bewegungsstörungen bei akuter Bulbocapninvergiftung. Arch. f. exper. Path. u. Pharmakol. **103:** 1, 1924.

SCHALTENBRAND, G. Gibt es eine Scopolaminsucht bei Parkinsonismuskranken? Med. Klin. **20:** 176, 1924.

SCHARF, J. H. Genoscopolamine; its use in Parkinsonism. J. Nerv. & Ment. Dis. **89:** 682, 1939.

SCHEIFFARTH, F. Die Therapie extrapyramidaler Bewegungsstörungen. Fortschr. d. Therap. **15:** 524, 1939.

SCHEIFFARTH, F. Belladonna-Vollextrakte in der Enzephalitistherapie. Deutsche med. Wchnschr. **66:** 318, 1940.

SCHLEZINGER, N. S., AND ALPERS, B. J. The use of syntropan in Parkinsonism. Am. J. M. Sc. **210:** 374, 1941.

SCHMITZ, A. Erfahrungen bei der Behandlung der chronischen Encephalitis mit der Bulgarischen Kur (Homburg 680). Psychiat.-neurol. Wchnschr. **41:** 146, 1939.

SCHROEDER, K. Sulfosin treatment of general paralysis and other disorders. Lancet 1929, II, 1081.

SCHROEDER, K. Ueber die Sulfosinbehandlung von nichtsyphilitischen Zentralnervensystem-Erkrankungen. . . . Deutsche med. Wchnschr. **55:** 1711, 1929.

SCHUSTER, J. Über das zwangsweise Brüllen als hyperkinetisches Symptom des Parkinsonismus. Klin. Wchnschr. **4:** 1824, 1925.

SCHUSTER, P. Ergebnisse von Banisterinversuchen an Nervenkranken. Med. Klin. **25:** 562, 1929.

SCHUSTER, P. Hat sich das Harmin bei der Behandlung des Parkinsonismus bewährt? Deutsche med. Wchnschr. **57:** 1537, 1931.

SECKBACH, M. Erfolgreiche Behandlung des Parkinsonismus und der Paralysis agitans mit "Eustateina." Med. Klin. **27:** 1218, 1931.

SEPP, E. K., and others. Die Oxytherapie bei der epidemischen Encephalitis. Arch. f. Psychiat. **81:** 61, 1927.

SHAPIRO, M. J. Benzedrine in treatment of narcolepsy. Minnesota Med. **20:** 28, 1937.

SHAPIRO, S. Treatment of Parkinsonian states by Juster's method; report of 23 cases. J. Nerv. & Ment. Dis. **68:** 488, 1928.

SIEGMUND, H. Anatomisch nachgewiesene Folgen von Tonus- und Motilitätsstörungen des Verdauungskanals bei Enzephalitikern die mit Atropin behandelt werden. München. med. Wchnschr. **82:** 453, 1935.

SILVESTRI. Il tartaro stibiato nella ençefalite epidemica. Riforma med. **39:** 898, 1923.

SKILLERN, P. G. Tic of diaphragm (postencephalitic) relieved by resection of phrenic nerves. J. A. M. A. **96:** 2098, 1931.

SOLDI, A., AND TRABUCCHI, C. Le radici di Atropa Belladonna nella cura del parkinsonismo encefalitico. Policlinico (sez. prat.) **43:** 2051, 1936.

SOLOMON, P., MITCHELL, R. S., AND PRINZMETAL, M. The use of benzedrine sulfate in postencephalitic Parkinson's disease. J. A. M. A. **108:** 765, 1937.

SOUQUES, A. Les syndromes parkinsoniens. Presse méd. **29:** 524, 1921.

SOUQUES, A. Traitement des syndromes parkinsoniens par les injections intraveineuses de liquide céphalo-rachidien de malade. Bull. et mém. Soc. d. hôp. de Paris **46:** 1736, 1922.

SOUQUES, A., AND MOUQUIN. Inefficacité du traitement des syndromes parkinsoniens postencéphalitiques par les injections intraveineuses de liquide céphalo-rachidien de malade. Rev. neurol. **39:** 1356, 1922.

STAEHELIN, J. E. Die postenzephalitischen Affektstörungen. Schweiz. Arch. f. Neurol. u. Psychiat. **14:** 131, 1924.

STARK, H. Neuer Vorschlag zur Encephalitisbehandlung. Arch. f. Psychiat. u. Nervenkr. **96:** 770, 1932.

STEEN, P. Stramonium in chronic epidemic encephalitis. New York State J. Med. **31:** 1090, 1931.

STEFANI, S. Piroterapia spontanea malarico-tifica in parkinsoniano postencefalitico. Rassegna di studi psichiat. **17:** 656, 1928.

STEMPLINGER, F. Zur Therapie des postenzephalitischen Parkinsonismus. München med. Wchnschr. **73:** 1930, 1926.

STERN, F. Epidemische Encephalitis. In: Handbuch der Neurologie. XIII, 307. Berlin, 1936.

STERN, F. Sanokrysin bei Erkrankungen des Zentralnervensystems. Deutsche med. Wchnschr. **59:** 935, 1933.

STERNBERG, E. Ueber die Behandlung des Parkinsons und ähnlicher Zuztandsbilder mit Stramonium. Nervenarzt **3:** 3, 1930.

STERN-PIPER, L. Blutsenkungsgeschwindigkeit und postencephalitische Störungen. Ztschr. f. d. ges. Neurol. u. Psychiat. **91:** 633, 1924.

STEWART, W. B., AND EVANS, M. J. Preliminary notes on bacteriologic studies and treatment of chronic epidemic encephalitis. Am. J. M. Sc. **180:** 256, 1930.

STIEFLER, G. Narkolepsie nach Enzephalitis lethargica. Wien. klin. Wchnschr. **37:** 1044, 1924.

STIEFLER, G. Ueber die Sulfosinbehandlung bei Nerven- und Geisteskrankheiten. Psychiat.-neurol. Wchnschr. **31:** 347, 1929.

STRANSKY, E. Behandlungsversuche mit Koffein (kombiniert mit Vakzine) beim Parkinsonismus. Psychiat.-neurol. Wchnschr. **33:** 377, 1931.

STRAUCH. Die Bulgarische Kur bei Encephalitis chronica epidemica lethargica. Psychiat.-neurol. Wchnschr. **41:** 140, 1939.

SZYSZKA, W. Atropinbehandlung bei Parkinsonianismus. München. med. Wchnschr. **70:** 47, 1923.

TACHIBANA, S., AND HASUO, H. Über die Röntgenbestrahlung bei Encephalitis epidemica Typus B. Abstr. in: Zentralbl. f. d. ges. Neurol. u. Psychiat. **80:** 649, 1936.

TAYLOR, S. A., AND HOBART, F. G. Bulgarian belladonna. Pharm. J. **141:** 49, 1938.

TRAUTMANN, E., AND PANSDORF, H. Versuch einer Röntgenbestrahlung der chronischen Encephalitis. Klin. Wchnschr. **9:** 1444, 1930.

TREVES, M., AND TREVES, G. Il metronomo come mezzo di una delle turbie di linguaggio nella encefalite letargica. Riv. sper. di freniat. **58:** 1521, 1934.

TRIPI, G. Trattamento stricnico nei postencefalitici sottoposti a cura di atropa belladonna. Pisani **57:** 243, 1937.

URBINO. Le traitement du parkinsonism par l'extrait de racine de belladonne. Bruxelles méd. **17:** 1256, 1937.

VAN DER HORST, L. Bulgarian cure (belladonna) in parkinsonism. Nederl. tijdschr. v. geneesk. **83:** 3497, 1939.

VAN DER MEULEN, F. Its over de Gevaren van de Atropinkuur met hooge Doses. . . . Nederl. tijdschr. v. geneesk. **77:** 5693, 1933.

VAN DER WIELEN, P. De Bulgaarsche belladonnawortel. Nederl. tijdschr. v. geneesk. **82:** 24 (English summary 27), 1938.

VEDEL, PUECH, AND PAGES. Quelques résultats du traitement des syndromes parkinsoniens post-encéphalitiques par le salicylate de soude. Bull. Soc. d. sc. méd. et biol. de Montpellier **6:** 159, 1924–25.

VINCENT, AND DE MARTEL. Sympathectomie cervico-thoracique dans les syndromes parkinsoniens postencéphalitiques. Soc. neurol., Paris. April, 1925.

VOLLMER, H. The Bulgarian treatment of post-encephalitic Parkinsonism. J. Mt. Sinai Hosp. **6:** 93, 1939–40.

VOLLMER, H. Bulgarian treatment of Parkinson's disease. Arch. Neurol. & Psychiat. **43:** 1057, 1940.

VOR DER BRÜCK, G. Die Röntgenbestrahlung des Stammhirns und ihre Ergebnisse bei chronischer Encephalitis epidemica. Psychiat.-neurol Wchnschr. **41:** 305, 1939.

WERTHEIMER, P. Les possibilités chirurgicales dans la maladie de Parkinson. Presse méd. **33:** 1318, 1925.

VON WIESER, W. Weitere Erfahrungen mit der Röntgentherapie bei psychiatrischen und neurologischen Erkrankungen: Folgezustände bei Encephalitis epidemica. Strahlentherapie **33:** 380, 1929.

WINKLER. Zur Therapie der Encephalitis epidemica. Klin. Wchnschr. **6:** 1508, 1927.
1938.

VON WITZLEBEN, H. D. Chronisch rezidivierende Encephalitis. Arch. f. Psychiat. u. Nervenkr. **88:** 149, 1929.

von Witzleben, H. D. Die Behandlung der chronischen Encephalitis epidemica mit der bulgarischen Kur (Vorläufige Mitteilung). Psychiat.-neurol. Wchnschr. **39:** 403, 1937.

von Witzleben, H. D. Die Behandlung der post-enzephalitischen Hypersomnie mit Ephedrin (Ephetonin). Therap. d. Gegenw. **78:** 475, 1937.

von Witzleben, H. D. Die Behandlung der chronischen Encephalitis epidemica (Parkinsonismus) mit der bulgarischen Kur. Klin. Wchnschr. **17:** 329, 369, 1938.

von Witzleben, H. D. Die Behandlung der chronischen Encephalitis epidemica mit der bulgarischen Kur. Schweiz. med. Wchnschr. **68:** 1352, 1938.

von Witzleben, H. D. Bulgarian treatment of postencephalitic Parkinsonism. Illinois J. Psychiat. 1, 1941.

von Witzleben, H. D. Ergebnisse der Behandlung des postencephalitischen Parkinsonismus mit Belladonna-Wurzelextract (Bulgakur). Schweiz. med. Wchnschr. **71:** 1941, no. 41.

von Witzleben, H. D., and Haufe, R. Richtlinien für die Uebungs- und Gymnastikbehandlung des postencephalitischen Parkinsonismus. Schweiz. med. Wchnschr. **70:** 978, 1940.

von Witzleben, H. D., and Werner, A. Encephalitis epidemica, Hirntumor, Multiple Sklerose. Nervenarzt **12:** 78, 1939.

von Witzleben, H. D., and Werner, A. Behandlung der chronischen Encephalitis epidemica (Parkinsonismus). Bulgarische Kur mit "Homburg 680." Deutsche med. Wchnschr. **64:** 1174, 1938.

Worster-Drought, C., and Hill, T. R. The treatment of chronic encephalitic Parkinsonism with dried preparations of stramonium. Lancet 1930, I, 1225.

Wuite, J. Die Hirsauer Behandelingsmethode van het postencephalitisch Parkinsonisme. Groningen theses, 1924. (English summary p. 126.)

Yoshida, K. [Untersuchung über den Skelettmuskeltonus. V Mitteilung. Über die Lumbalanästhesie und Narkose bei Parkinsonismus]. Acta scholae med. univ. imp. in Kioto **17:** 395, 1935. Abstr. in: Zentralbl. f. d. ges. Neurol. u. Psychiat. **77:** 231, 1935.

Yoshida, K., and Imai, M. [Untersuchungen über den Skelettmuskeltonus. VI Mitteilung. Vergleichung der Wirkung des Atropins mit der des Scopolamins auf den Rigor.] Acta scholae med. univ. imp. in Kioto **17:** 404, 1935. Abstr. in: Zentralbl. f. d. ges. Neurol. u. Psychiat. **77:** 231, 1935.

YOUNG, D., AND SCOVILLE, W. B. Paranoid psychosis in narcolepsy and the possible danger of benzedrine therapy. M. Clin. N. Amer. **22:** 637, 1938.

ZAHORSKI. Günstiger Einfluss hoher Skopolamindosen auf den Parkinsonismus. Abstr. in: Zentralbl. f. d. ges. Neurol. u. Psychiat. **40:** 200, 1925.

ZISKIND, E., AND SOMMERFELD-ZISKIND, E. Phenobarbital contraindicated in parkinsonism. J. A. M. A. **109:** 20, 1937.

ZISKIND, E., AND SOMMERFELD-ZISKIND, E. Metrazol therapy in chronic encephalitis with parkinsonism; effect on oculogyric crises. Bull. Los Angeles Neurol. Soc. **3:** 186, 1938.

ZUCKER, K. Ueber die Wirkung des Physostigmins bei Erkrankungen des extrapyramidalen Systems. Monatschr. f. Psychiat. **58:** 11, 1925.